Pre-Diabetes

Cookbook

Over 200 Easy, Delicious & Proven Insulin Resistance Recipes to Reverse Prediabetes and Diabetes. 30 Day Action Plan & Exercises Included.

Author: Sandra Williams

Special Bonus

Ready to receive over 600 Delicious & Easy Recipes for FREE?

We want to thank you for purchasing the book and we hope to make your belly happy with the recipes that follow. As a token of our appreciation we have a little gift for you.

We are a team of small but passionate cookbook writers and our mission is to make cooking fun, simple and delicious. Writing recipes gives us a chance to have fun, be creative and let other people know that healthy and delicious food does not have to be complicated nor take hours and hours.

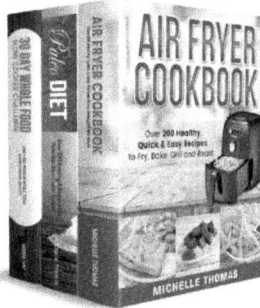

Only sign up for the cookbook box set if you are ready to be absolutely amazed with over 600 proven, delicious and easy to make recipes.

To access the gift page type in www.bit.ly/2Ho82AH or email us at info@limitlessrecipes.com to get the box set delivered to your email.

Limitless Recipes
Like us on Facebook and join our private Facebook group community for more recipes and gifts.
@limitlessrecipes
Follow us on Instagram
Limitless Recipes
Follow us on Pinterest.

Want to be a part of our closed Facebook group?
We are working on building an engaged community discussing recipes and healthy eating in our closed Facebook group. If you would like to be involved in the discussions about cooking, what is working, what is not working and receive information about gifts and promotions, we would be delighted to add you.

Type in Limitless Recipes on Facebook or write us at info@limitlessrecipes.com. Come say hi!

Happy Cooking!

Table of Contents

Introduction

Wouldn't it be amazing if our bodies gave us some form of warning to let us know when we were approaching unhealthy territories like the backup warnings on our car system? Well the truth is it does! Sure, it doesn't beep uncontrollably as a sign of warning but it does throw us a few warning flares to let us now it is time to take precautions to avoid further dangers. This is exactly what Prediabetes does.

The term prediabetes refers to state in which our bodies face higher than normal blood glucose levels that are not yet at the level for it to be called type 2 diabetes. For those of us who understand blood sugar level readings this would be around 7.0 mmol/L in fasting plasma or 6.5% or higher in A1C. The upside of prediabetes is that not every person who develops prediabetes will necessarily progress into type 2 diabetes, but there is a high possibility especially if you do not head to the warning signs that your body is throwing out to you.

Due to this, it is incredibly important that you not only head the warning signs but also start becoming informed on the risk factors and changes you will be required to make in your lifestyle to halt the onset of type 2 diabetes.

Identify Risks for Developing Type 2 Diabetes

As with every other ailment in life, prediabetes can sneak up on you so it is vital that you remain educated and get the proper checks required on a regular basis. Even more so if you suffer from other high-risk factors or the "metabolic syndrome". What this means is that you find that you are also suffering from hypertension, high cholesterol or have gain a lot of excess fat around your waist.

The need for testing more frequently also increases as you become older so people below the age of 40 gets the luxury of testing minimally as they see fit while as you approach or surpass 40 the testing requirement increases to at least once every 3 years. The onus is therefore on you to listen to your body and determine if it is flashing you signs of the common risk factors mentioned above so that you can increase the frequency of your screening if needed.

How to Stay Motivated, Manage Stress & How to Track Your Progress

As you can imagine getting yourself stressed out will only make the likelihood of you developing a more serious condition even higher so it is vital that you figure out ways in which to remain motivated on getting better when you find out that you have prediabetes, manage your stress levels and keep track of how you are cooping. Here are a few tips that may help you to achieve this:

Try to keep eating healthy
It's a known fact that whenever stress takes over healthy eating habits get thrown out the window. But in order to remain on the right track back to being healthy you will have to make a conscious effect to only eat meals that are not only balanced but healthy. So, try to substitute those take out boxes for fresh fruits and vegetables as these will not only build help rebuild your immune system bet also keep you fuller for longer without binge eating.

Try to remain active
When trying to maintain a healthier lifestyle, taking time out to get some exercise in is vital. It has been proven over the years that simple exercises such as yoga, jogging or lifting weights can significantly ease stress and improve your mood. It can also serve as a distraction from all the other things going on in your life and allow you to center yourself and focus more on the positives of life.

I recommend you to buy any of these exercising equipment that will help you ease your stress and improve your mood: Resistance Bands (Link to Amazon: https://amzn.to/2Tsx6IN), Body Rider Exercise Upright Fan Bike (Link to Amazon: https://amzn.to/2OjDHUN) and Stamina Pro Ab/Hyper Bench (Link to Amazon: https://amzn.to/2YdfDYc).

Here are some pre-diabetes supplements that I have personally used not just to avoid diabetes but to also enhance my mood and to stay motivated while doing the diet. Diabetic Support Supplement (Link to Amazon: https://amzn.to/2UQ94sz). Probiotic (Link to Amazon: https://amzn.to/2HCzNpl) and Biotin (Link to Amazon: https://amzn.to/2CznQwJ).

How to Make and Fast Delicious Recipes Without Fancy and Expensive Ingredients

While it might be fine to spend a bit on a few kitchen staples, there are many more ingredients you could just as easily craft on your kitchen table with sheer creativity and some work. Here are a few hacks you should note if you want to run a budget-friendly kitchen that you can actually afford.

Buttermilk
There are a few ingredients that always seem to be missing when you actually crave them, and one of such is buttermilk. Before you waste money in the store and on gas for your car when next you crave for some biscuits or pancakes, use this hack as a more affordable alternative.

Cake and Self-Rising Flour
I personally don't see why you should need these, but then, if these are your kind of snacks and you need to have them, by all means go ahead. To save cost on this, you would have to do more than replacing regular ole' AP here. What you need is an easy-to-follow hack that you can make with cornstarch, a bit of baking powder and, some salt. This guide will help you discover how to combine these to create that amazing cake.

Hack Your Alcohol Cabinet
instead of cutting deep into your wallet by buying alcohol in bars, a much smarter way is to create yours. For just a few dollars, you could infuse your own drinks with the aid of simple mixers, and produce drinks that taste as if you spent $20 to get them at a bar. What if you don't want to go all hardcore? You could simply take your apple peels headed for the bin, and put them to good use by infusing your bourbon. You won't even need a mixer for this, yet the result would be so spectacular.

Seasonal Availability when Purchasing Foods

Just like the changes in weather across the globe, fresh produce come and go. With different seasons come different array of fresh produce. There is no better time to experiment and try out new recipes. You can even decide to rework some of those old, boring ones and see what you could get out of them by incorporating more of the seasonal fruits and vegetables. Not only will this stun your palate, there are so many health benefits for your body too. Here are a few of the benefits of eating seasonally!

Seasonal Produce:
- Is Cheaper
- Tastes Better
- Is Fresher
- Has Higher Nutritional Value
- Is More Environmentally-Friendly
- Is Free from Overseas Contaminants

Let's quickly make a really important note that there are times when it is nearly impossible to get local and seasonal produces. This is alright. The really important thing here is that you keep making deliberate decisions to go for them wherever and whenever possible. Eating seasonal and local produces are really important decisions for your health and your wallet.

How to Seamlessly Incorporate Prediabetes Diet into Your Lifestyle

While there are some risk factors about prediabetes that are hard to control, many of them could still be effectively mitigated, if attended to. With some adjustments to your lifestyle, you could keep your blood sugar levels balanced, while staying within a healthy weight.

Look out for carbs with high glycemic index
The glycemic index (GI) is an effective tool used to determine the level of effect a particular food could have on your blood sugar.

When you consume foods with high glycemic index (GI), they would make your blood sugar level spike faster. On the other end, if the foods you consume are ranked lower on that scale, the effect they would have on your blood sugar level would be less. Foods that have high fiber are usually low on the glycemic index (GI), while foods that have been processed and refined, with little nutrients and fiber contents are usually high on the GI. If you want what is best for your blood sugar, stick to foods that are low on the GI. These are a few examples that you can incorporate into your diet:

- beans
- stone-ground whole wheat bread
- steel-cut oats (not those instant oatmeal)
- sweet potatoes
- corn
- non-starchy vegetables, like carrots and field greens
- pasta (preferably whole wheat)

Portion control
An effective way to keep your diet low on GI is to practice good portion control. What this means is that you should limit how much food you eat in one sitting. Most times in the United States, portions are much larger than what the serving sizes are intended to be. Take a bagel serving size, for example. Even though it is only about a half, many people would eat the whole bagel as a serving.

If you want to really determine how much goes into your mouth, a good place to start is on the food labels. You will find listed on the label how much calories, carbohydrates, proteins, fat, and other nutrition information a serving of a particular food contains.

Eat more foods rich in fiber
There are so many benefits that fiber offers your body. First, It helps you feel fuller for a longer period. The bulk that fiber adds to your diet helps make your bowel movements easier. By eating fiber-rich foods, you are less likely to overeat. These fiber-rich foods will also prevent you from experiencing the "crash" that usually follows the consumption of high-sugar foods. These high-sugar foods will only give you an energy boost for a short while, before fizzling out and making you feel tired.

Some of these high-fiber foods are:
- whole-grain breads
- beans and legumes
- whole grain cereals
- whole grains such as quinoa or barley

- fruits and vegetables with edible skin
- whole wheat pasta

Metabolism- Boosting Exercises

The job of your metabolism sounds pretty simple: It helps in regulating the conversion rate of the food you eat into the energy your body uses. However, even though metabolism sounds simple, there is more to it than that. Indeed, an increase in your metabolism would translate to weight loss. But our bodies differ, and we don't all experience metabolisms at the same rate. For some people, it is faster, while some others have it slower. Even your base metabolic rate— that is, the amount of calories you would burn lying on your back all day without doing anything—varies from person to the other, depending on such factors as your weight and bone density.

If you would like to boost your metabolism yourself, these are a few to help you achieve that:

Fire-Feet Drill:
Start this exercise by keeping your feet wider than your shoulders. Allow your knees to bend slightly and keep your hips right behind you. While resting on the balls of your feet, start running in place as quick as you can, as if the floor is hot. After about 10 seconds each round, do either a jump squat (if you are a beginner) or a tuck jump (if you are an expert) as high as you can. Now return straight to your fire feet again.

Jumping Knee Up-Downs:
Start this in the base of your squat by taking a step back into a reverse lunge, and lowering your knee till it touches the floor. After this, bring your other knee low to the floor. Step one feet back up first, and then the other. Then, end this with an explosive jump which would get you right back down again to the base of your squat, just as in the beginning. Do this repeatedly.

Mountain Climbers:
Begin in a pushup-plank position. Make sure to place your hands firmly on the floor, directly under your shoulders. Ensure that your hips remain parallel to the ground, with your feet back and together. In rapid succession, run your knees straight towards your chest without touching it, alternating your legs each rep. Throughout the exercise, keep your shoulders right over your wrists and prevent your hips from raising.

30 Day Action Plan

To start this plan of action, I recommend you to use a food diary. Here are some you can choose from BookFactory Food Journal (Link to Amazon: https://amzn.to/2YdftQx) DIETMINDER Personal Food & Fitness Journal (link to Amazon: https://amzn.to/2OldzZI) and Daily Food Intake Journal (Link to Amazon: https://amzn.to/2HBMvoG).

Day 1 – Day 3: Set a weight loss goal

Weight loss is a noble pursuit, but a lot of people have blown it way out of proportion. You don't have to set a crazy weight loss goal. You don't have to be dramatic about it at all to notice significant impact. All it takes it a few pounds at first. If you are overweight, losing just 7% of your total body weight could be all you need to start stabilizing your blood sugar level. This would be around 20 to 30 pounds for someone who weighs around 300 pounds.

Day 4 - Day 6: Track Your Food Consumption with A Food Journal

for any weight loss plan to work, a healthy, low-calorie meal plan has to be strictly followed. This is an essential ingredient of the process. To properly evaluate the quality and quantity of the food you consume, you must start tracking everything that goes into your mouth, from meals and snacks to that cup of beverages and the quick bites here and there. If you manage to keep track for just a few days, you will be surprised by and be able to recognize some worrisome patterns and bad habits you've been cultivating.

Day 7 – Day 10: Start making smarter food choices

Do not confuse a prediabetes diagnosis to mean that you have to eliminate entire food groups or starve all day. On the contrary, you can still eat fine. All you have to do is to start with one small change. It could start with a meal or even a snack. To lose a few extra pounds without burning out, all it takes is a small change. So:
- Reduce your portions of foods high in calories, sugar and fat.
- In place of the less-healthy food choices you've been making, try out a few healthier foods.
- Go for foods that have lower saturated fat, trans-fat and added sugars.
- Replace your sugar-sweetened beverages like energy drinks, soda, and juice with cleaner ones like water or tea.

Day 11 – Day 13: Stick to a healthy fat and calorie range

We all have our different needs. To tailor these tips and guidelines to your unique needs, you should work hand-in-hand with your doctor or your diabetes prevention specialist. Remember to read the nutrition facts labels carefully and track your daily food consumption, to make sure that you're still staying right in your target range.

Day 14 – Day 17: Find little ways to move more

We don't all have hours to spend at a gym or daily. However, don't let that be an excuse not to move your muscles. There are many ways to get your muscles moving throughout the day. Even as little as 30 minutes of moderate exercises, like brisk walking, four or five days a week has been proven to aid in weight loss and blood sugar levels management.

Day 18 – Day 21: Quit smoking and drop other bad habits

According to the Centers for Disease Control and Prevention (CDC), there is as high as 30 to 40 percent greater risk of smokers developing Type 2 diabetes than their non-smoking counterparts. Smoking is dangerous on so many levels. It can cause inflammation and interfere with normal cell function, which can eventually lead to diabetes. In addition, smokers have been found to have higher amounts of cortisol, a hormone known to elevate blood sugar levels.

Day 22 – Day 25: Double up on your support systems

Sometimes, we need a little bit of extra help and support at different stages of life. Make sure you look into online diabetes tools which can prove helpful as you keep moving along this journey. Diabetes HealthSense is one of such example. It assists you in creating a customized plan that fits into your new lifestyle. If you need to find more general information, you can always get them from the National Diabetes Prevention Program, or simply locate a diabetes prevention program closest to you.

Day 26 – Day 30: Stay in touch with your doctor

After a prediabetes diagnosis, resist any urge to battle this in isolation. Maintaining your communication regularly with your healthcare professional is more important than ever at this stage. As you strive towards cultivating better and more wholesome eating and exercise habits, your doctor will most likely want to keep track of your blood sugar levels or even adjust or downright change your medications to make sure that they stay in a healthy range.

Now that you are equipped with all this knowledge about the prediabetes diet, it is time to dive into some delicious recipes!

PREDIABETES SALADS, SAUCES & SALAD DRESSINGS

1. Balsamic Hummus Salad Dressing

Ingredients

5 Tablespoons hummus
4 Tablespoons balsamic vinegar
2 Tablespoons extra-virgin olive oil

1 teaspoon garlic powder
sea salt and pepper to taste

Directions

In a small bowl, whisk all ingredients until combined. Serve over tossed greens and vegetables

Serves: 4	Prep Time: 15 mins.		Cooking Time: 0 mins.
Calories: 70	Protein: 1g	Carbs: 3g	Fat: 7g

2. Creamy Avocado Salad Dressing

Ingredients

1 ripe avocado, pitted, peeled and chopped
½ cup extra-virgin olive oil
Lime juice from 1 lime
3 Tablespoons freshly squeezed orange juice

½ teaspoon minced chives
1 Tablespoon cilantro, finely chopped
sea salt and pepper to taste

Directions

In a blender, puree all ingredients until smooth. Serve over tossed greens and vegetables.

Serves: 4	Prep Time: 15 mins.		Cooking Time: 0 mins.
Calories: 38.2	Protein: 0.8g	Carbs: 3.6g	Fat: 2.6g

3. Creamy Lemon Herb Salad Dressing

Ingredients

1/2 cup hemp hearts
juice of 1 lemon
1 Tablespoon. chopped cilantro
1 small garlic clove, coarsely chopped

1 teaspoon minced chives
1 Tablespoon chopped dill
sea salt and pepper to taste

Directions

In a blender, puree all ingredients until smooth. If needed, add water for a thinner consistency. Serve over tossed greens and vegetables.

Serves: 4	Prep Time: 15 mins.		Cooking Time: 0 mins.
Calories: 121.5	Protein: 17g	Carbs: 0.5g	Fat: 5.2g

4. Cold Asian Noodle Salad

Ingredients

sesame oil, 1 teaspoon
rice wine vinegar, 2 tbsps.
Peanuts, 4 tbsps., unsalted, for garnish
1 tbsp. hoisin sauce
3 tbsps. soy sauce
1 teaspoon hot chili oil
5 tbsps. extra-virgin olive oil
celery stalks, 2, julienned
carrot, 1, thinly sliced

cilantro leaves, 3 tbsps., minced
soba noodles, 1 package
Napa cabbage, 1/2 cup, thinly sliced
green onions, 5 stalks, thinly sliced
red bell pepper, 1/2 , julienned
bok choy, 1/2 cup, julienned
bean sprouts, 1 cup, optional
sesame seeds, 3 tbsps. , toasted, for garnish

Directions

Boil water in a medium stock pot, add salt and cook noodles. When this finish, transfer your noodles to an ice bath so it can cool down quickly. Drain and set aside. Mix together your olive oil, hoisin, chili oil, soy sauce, vinegar, and sesame oil in a bowl. Add in all your noodle and prepared vegetables. Garnish with sesame seeds and peanuts, if desired.

Serves: 4	Prep Time: 15 mins.		Cooking Time: 7 mins.
Calories: 200.3	Protein: 13.5g	Carbs: 20.2g	Fat: 8.3g

5. Faux Potato Salad

Ingredients

1-pound cauliflower
1/3 cup plain yogurt
1 Tablespoon olive oil
2 Tablespoon white vinegar
1 Tablespoon Dijon mustard
1 teaspoon garlic powder
1/4 teaspoon paprika

1/4 teaspoon celery salt
1/4 teaspoon sea salt
1/4 teaspoon pepper
2 eggs hard boiled, chopped
1/4 cup chopped red onion
1/4 cup chopped scallions

Directions

Set your cauliflower to steam for about 10 minutes (you want it to be fork tender). Cool to room temperature for 20-30 minutes. If you prefer the taste of roasted cauliflower, go for it! For the dressing, place the next 9 ingredients in a bowl and whisk until well combined. Stir the dressing into the cauliflower and add in onion, eggs and scallions. Place to chill until you are ready to serve.

Serves: 4	Prep Time: 15 mins.		Cooking Time: 7 mins.
Calories: 94.3	Protein: 3.1g	Carbs: 3.8g	Fat: 7.4g

6. Shrimp, Zucchini, and Wilted Kale Noodle Salad

Ingredients

2 Tablespoon extra virgin olive oil
4 cloves garlic, minced
8 ounces deveined shrimp, tails removed
1 bunch organic kale, stems removed, chopped
(about 6 cups)
1 teaspoon salt

1/2 teaspoon pepper
1-pint cherry tomatoes
2 cups zucchini noodles
Juice of 2 lemons (about 1/2 cup)
1/4 cup fresh basil, chopped

Directions

Set your oil to get hot over medium heat in a large skillet. Add garlic and cook just until soft. Add shrimp and cook until curled around edges and both sides are pink. Lower the heat then add in your tomatoes, salt, pepper and kale. Continue to cook until kale is wilted. Stir in lemon juice and zucchini noodles and cook for 2-3 more minutes until zucchini is firm/tender. Serve topped with fresh basil.

Serves: 4   **Prep Time: 15 mins.**   **Cooking Time: 7 mins.**
Calories: 94.3   **Protein: 3.1g**   **Carbs: 3.8g**   **Fat: 7.4g**

7. Mexican Cole Slaw

Ingredients

Bottom of Form
8 cups thinly sliced green cabbage
4 cups thinly sliced red cabbage
(You can use all green or all red cabbage, if you prefer)
4 green onions, thinly sliced
1 cup chopped cilantro (or more)

8 Tablespoons plain yogurt
6 Tablespoons fresh lime juice (more or less to taste)
hot sauce to taste (about 1 teaspoon Tabasco sauce is good)
salt to taste

Directions

Add your cilantro, onions and cabbage to a salad bowl. In a small bowl, whisk together, yogurt, lime juice, and hot sauce. Use a wooden spoon to fold dressing into cabbage mixture. Finish with a dash of salt and serve or chill.

Serves: 8   **Prep Time: 15 mins.**   **Cooking Time: 0 mins.**
Calories: 91.9   **Protein: 3.5g**   **Carbs: 17.2g**   **Fat: 2.5g**

Entrees

8. Ranch-Style Dressing

Ingredients

3/4 cup non-fat yogurt

1/4 cup fat-free mayonnaise

1 tbsp white or cider vinegar

1/2 tsp sugar

2 tsp Dijon mustard

1 green onion, finely minced

1 clove garlic, crushed

1/4 tsp dried thyme

freshly ground pepper

Directions

Measure all ingredients into a small bowl. Mix well and refrigerate. Serve chilled. Stir before using.

Serves: 10	Prep Time: 15 mins.		Cooking Time: 0 mins.
Calories: 9	Protein: 1g	Carbs: 1g	Fat: 0.1g

9. Simply Basic Vinaigrette

Ingredients

1/4 cup olive or canola oil

1/4 cup rice, balsamic or red wine vinegar

1/4 cup chicken or vegetable broth

1 tsp Dijon mustard

1 tbsp honey or maple syrup

1/2 tsp dried basil (or 1 tbsp fresh minced)

1 clove garlic, crushed

salt and freshly ground pepper, to taste

Directions

Combine all ingredients and mix well. Drizzle over your favorite salad greens and toss to mix.

Serves: 12	Prep Time: 15 mins.		Cooking Time: 0 mins.
Calories: 43	Protein: 1g	Carbs: 1g	Fat: 4.1g

10. Barley Salad with Honey Mustard Dressing

Ingredients:

3 cup lightly salted water

1 cup pearl or pot barley (if using pot barley, soak it overnight)

1 red pepper, chopped

4 green onions, chopped

1/2 cup Honey Mustard Dressing

2–3 tbsp fresh dill and/or basil, minced

2 tbsp toasted sunflower seeds, optional

Directions:

Bring water to a boil. Add barley and simmer covered for 45 to 60 minutes, until tender. (Pearl barley takes 45 minutes to cook; pot barley takes about an hour.) Drain if necessary. Barley can be cooked in advance and refrigerated up to 24 hours. Combine chilled barley with remaining ingredients and toss to mix. Add a little lemon juice to moisten.

Serves: 6	Prep Time: 10 mins.		Cooking Time: 10 mins.
Calories: 179	Protein: 4g	Carbs: 34g	Fat: 4g

11. Lighter Caesar Salad Dressing

Ingredients:

1/2 cup non-fat yogurt
1/4 cup fat-free or low-fat mayonnaise
1 clove garlic, crushed
1/4 cup grated Parmesan cheese

1/2 tsp Worcestershire sauce
2 tbsp lemon juice (to taste)
3/4 tsp salt (to taste)
freshly ground pepper, to taste

Ingredients:

Combine all ingredients and mix well; chill. Delicious over Romaine lettuce or spinach.
Yield: about 1 cup. Dressing will keep 4 or 5 days in the refrigerator.

Serves: 10	Prep Time: 15 mins.		Cooking Time: 0 mins.
Calories: 15	Protein: 1g	Carbs: 2g	Fat: 0.6g

12. Balsamic Salad Splash

Ingredients:

1/4 cup balsamic vinegar
1/4 cup water
1/4 cup honey

1/4 tsp garlic powder
3–4 drops Tabasco sauce (to taste)
2 tsp olive or canola oil

Directions:

Combine all ingredients in a jar; shake well. Refrigerate until needed. Shake well before serving. Dressing can be stored in the refrigerator for up to a month.

Serves: 4	Prep Time: 10 mins.		Cooking Time: 0 mins.
Calories: 28	Protein: 0g	Carbs: 6g	Fat: 0.6g

13. Honey Mustard Dressing

Ingredients:

1/4 cup olive oil (preferably extra-virgin)
1/4 cup white or rice wine vinegar (or 2 tbsp
orange juice and 2 tbsp vinegar)
1/3 cup liquid honey

2 tbsp Dijon or prepared mustard
1/4 cup water
freshly ground pepper

Directions:

Add all your ingredients to a large enough jar, seal tightly and shake. Store in your refrigerator to be used within a month.

Serves: 1	Prep Time: 15 mins.		Cooking Time: 0 mins.
Calories: 42	Protein: 0g	Carbs: 5g	Fat: 2.7g

14. Orange Balsamic Vinaigrette

Ingredients

1/4 cup olive or canola oil
6 tbsp orange juice
1/4 cup balsamic vinegar
1–2 cloves garlic, crushed

2 tbsp minced fresh basil
1 tbsp sugar
salt and pepper, to taste

Directions

Combine all ingredients and mix well. Use as needed.

Serves: 6	Prep Time: 15 mins.		Cooking Time: 0 mins.
Calories: 43	Protein: 2g	Carbs: 1g	Fat: 3.7g

15. Shake It Up Salad Dressing

Ingredients

3/4 cup tomato or vegetable juice
3 tbsp balsamic or red wine vinegar
1 tbsp olive oil (preferably extra-virgin)
1–2 cloves garlic, crushed

1 tsp sugar (to taste)
1/2 tsp Worcestershire sauce (to taste)
1/2 tsp dry mustard
1/2 tsp dried basil

Directions

Measure all ingredients into a jar. Cover and shake well to blend. Refrigerate dressing. Shake well before serving. Serve over your favorite greens.

Serves: 10	Prep Time: 15 mins.		Cooking Time: 0 mins.
Calories: 14	Protein: 1g	Carbs: 1g	Fat: 0.9g

16. Dijon Mustard Sauce

Ingredients

2 tbsp Dijon mustard
2 tbsp fat-free or light mayonnaise
1 clove garlic, crushed

1/4 tsp Worcestershire sauce
3–4 drops of lemon juice

Directions

Combine all ingredients and mix to blend.

Serves: 2	Prep Time: 10 mins.		Cooking Time: 0 mins.
Calories: 14	Protein: 1g	Carbs: 2g	Fat: 0.6g

17.   Pre-diabetes Pesto

Ingredients

2 tbsp pine nuts (or walnuts)
2 cups tightly packed fresh basil leaves
1/2 cup fresh parsley
4 cloves garlic, peeled

2–3 tbsp grated Parmesan cheese
2 tbsp olive oil (extra-virgin is best)
1/4 cup tomato juice or vegetable broth
salt and pepper, to taste

Directions

Place nuts in a small skillet and brown over medium heat for 2 to 3 minutes. Wash basil and parsley; dry thoroughly. Start the food processor and drop garlic through feed tube. Process until minced. Add parm. cheese, parsley, basil and nuts. Process until fine. Top lightly with juice and oil slowly while processing and continue until fully blended. Season to taste.

Serves: 4	**Prep Time: 15 mins.**		**Cooking Time: 5 mins.**
Calories: 27	**Protein: 1g**	**Carbs: 1g**	**Fat: 2.4g**

18.   Cheater's Hi-Fiber Pasta Sauce

Ingredients

1 cup cooked lentils (or canned, rinsed and well-drained)
1 jar vegetarian spaghetti sauce (about 3 cups)

1/4 cup water
1–2 tbsp red or white wine, if desired

Directions

Process lentils in your food processor until puréed. Add spaghetti sauce and process until well mixed, scraping down sides of bowl as needed. Combine puréed mixture with water and wine (if using) in a large sauce pan. Bring to a boil and simmer partially covered for 10 minutes (or microwave uncovered on HIGH for 10 minutes), stirring occasionally.

Serves: 8	**Prep Time: 15 mins.**		**Cooking Time: 15 mins.**
Calories: 101	**Protein: 4g**	**Carbs: 15g**	**Fat: 3.7g**

19.   Quick 'n Easy Tomato Sauce

Ingredients:

28 oz can (796 ml) tomatoes (stewed, whole or crushed)
5-1/2 oz can (156 ml) tomato paste
1 tsp olive oil (preferably extra-virgin)
3 cloves garlic, crushed
salt and pepper, to taste

1/4 tsp cayenne or red pepper flakes
1/2 tsp oregano
1 tbsp fresh basil, minced (or 1/2 tsp dried)
1/2 tsp sugar
1–2 tbsp red or white wine, optional

Directions:

Allow your sauce to come a boil, then lower the heat so that it's just a simmer. Cover and allow to cook for about 25 minutes, while stirring on occasion. Adjust seasonings to taste.

Serves: 6	**Prep Time: 10 mins.**		**Cooking Time: 25 mins.**
Calories: 43	**Protein: 9g**	**Carbs: 9g**	**Fat: 0.8g**

20. Sun-Dried Tomato Pesto

Ingredients:

1/2 cup sun-dried tomatoes (dry-pack)
1/3 cup tightly packed fresh basil leaves
1/2 cup parsley
4–5 large cloves garlic

2 tbsp finely ground almonds
3 tbsp grated Parmesan cheese
2 tbsp olive oil (preferably extra-virgin)
1/2 cup tomato juice

Ingredients:

Cover sun-dried tomatoes with boiling water. Let stand for 20 minutes, until rehydrated. Drain well. Rinse basil and parsley; dry well. Allow your processor t start up then add in your garlic while running. Process until minced. Add sun-dried tomatoes, basil, parsley, almonds and Parmesan cheese. Process until fine, about 15 to 20 seconds. Add olive oil and tomato juice and process until well blended, scraping down sides of bowl as necessary.

Serves: 2	Prep Time: 10 mins.		Cooking Time: 20 mins.
Calories: 31	Protein: 1g	Carbs: 99g	Fat: 2.2g

21. Spaghetti with Roasted Tomato, Garlic and Basil Sauce

Ingredients:

Roasted Tomato, Garlic and Basil Sauce
1 lb (500 g) enriched spaghetti

Grated Parmesan cheese, optional

Directions:

Prepare sauce and keep it warm. Cook pasta according to package directions. Drain, reserving about 1/2 cup of the cooking water in the pot. Do not rinse pasta. Return pasta to the pot. Add just enough of the sauce to lightly coat the pasta; mix well. Place on serving plates. Serve with additional sauce. Sprinkle with a little grated Parmesan cheese, if desired.

Serves: 6	Prep Time: 10 mins.		Cooking Time: 7 mins.
Calories: 321	Protein: 16g	Carbs: 60g	Fat: 2.8g

22. Roasted Tomato, Garlic and Basil Sauce

Ingredients:

2 dozen Italian plum tomatoes (3 lb/1.4 kg)
2 onions, peeled
1 large red pepper, seeded
6–8 cloves garlic, peeled

1–2 tbsp extra-virgin olive oil
1/4–1/2 cup fresh basil, to taste salt and pepper, to taste

Directions:

Preheat oven to 400°F. Core tomatoes and cut in half lengthwise. Cut onions and red pepper into chunks. Arrange in a single layer on a non-stick baking sheet along with garlic. Drizzle lightly with oil. Roast uncovered at 400°F for 45 to 50 minutes, or until vegetables are soft and lightly browned.
Combine roasted vegetables with basil in the processor. (You may have to do this in 2 batches.) Process until smooth. Season to taste with salt and pepper.

Serves: 8	Prep Time: 10 mins.		Cooking Time: 50 mins.
Calories: 78	Protein: 2g	Carbs: 14g	Fat: 2.5g

23. Homemade Slow Cooker Ketchup

Ingredients

1 small onion, diced
2 granny smith apples, peeled and finely diced
2 cloves garlic, minced
½ teaspoon sea salt
1/4 teaspoon allspice
1/4 teaspoon cinnamon

1/8 teaspoon cloves
1/4 teaspoon ginger
2 tablespoons apple cider vinegar
1/4 cup water
6 oz. tomato paste

Directions

Combine all ingredients in a slow cooker. Set the cooker to low and let cook for 4 hours. Allow the mixture to cool slightly. Transfer to a blender and process the mix until smooth. Do not over-fill the container, as the warm ingredients will tend to expand and may splatter out. Once blended and silky smooth, place the ketchup into glass containers and allow it to come to room temperature before storing in the refrigerator.

Serves: 8	Prep Time: 15 mins.		Cooking Time: 5 mins.
Calories: 27	Protein: 1g	Carbs: 1g	Fat: 2.4g

24. Roasted Beet Hummus

Ingredients

1 ½ cups beets, peeled and chopped into ¼ inch dice
1 cup water
½ cup distilled white vinegar
Solution of 1 cup water and 1 cup white vinegar

1/4 cup rice wine vinegar
2 Tablespoons balsamic vinegar
1 small jalapeno, seeds included
1 red chili pepper
3 cloves garlic

Directions

Place chopped beet pieces into water/vinegar solution for up to 48 hours. After marinating, remove beets and add to 1 cup of boiling water. Let simmer for 15 minutes. If you prefer the taste of roasted beets, another option is to place beets in a pan and oven roast at 350° F for 35 minutes. Once cooked beets have cooled, place in a food processor or blender, add rice vinegar, balsamic vinegar, a jalapeno, chili pepper and garlic. Puree until smooth. If consistency is too thick, add some of the water-vinegar solution until it has a pleasing texture.

Yields: 1 ½ cups	Prep Time: 15 mins.		Cooking Time: 0 mins.
Calories: 75	Protein: 4g	Carbs: 1.5g	Fat: 5.3g

25. Cauliflower Hummus

Ingredients

1 head cauliflower (separated into florets, about 8 cups)
3/4 cup tahini
1/4 cup extra-virgin olive oil
3 Tablespoons lemon juice

6 cloves garlic
4 teaspoons cumin
1 ½ teaspoons sea salt
1 teaspoon paprika
1/4 teaspoon cayenne (optional)

Directions

Steam cauliflower florets for 5-7 minutes, until tender, but not limp. While the cauliflower is cooking, place tahini into a food processor and process until it is light and fluffy, about 2 minutes. Mash the garlic cloves, remove the skin, and cook in a small amount of olive oil over medium-high heat just for about 15-20 seconds, to release aroma. Remove from heat. Add the garlic to the food processor and pulse with the tahini until smooth. Place the steamed cauliflower florets into the food processor, a few at a time and process until it begins to look smooth. Add the rest of the ingredients, pulsing until well combined. Yield: about 4 cups

Serves: 10	**Prep Time: 15 mins.**	**Cooking Time: 0 mins.**
Calories: 67	**Protein: 2g**	**Carbs: 1.3g**	**Fat: 3.5g**

26. Artichoke Hummus

Ingredients

14oz. artichoke hearts, drained
1 clove garlic, minced
2 Tablespoons extra-virgin olive oil
1 Tablespoon fresh lemon juice
¼ cup tahini

¼ teaspoon ground cumin
Salt and pepper to taste
Finely minced fresh herbs such as parsley, basil, or oregano

Directions

Add drained artichoke hearts and minced garlic to the bowl of a food processor, process until coarsely chopped. Add olive oil, lemon juice, tahini, and ground cumin. Process again until mixture has a smooth texture. Season with salt and pepper to taste. Yield: 4 servings

Serves: 6	**Prep Time: 20 mins.**	**Cooking Time: 0 mins.**
Calories: 84	**Protein: 1.5g**	**Carbs: 1g**	**Fat: 4g**

27. No-Sugar Italian Marinara Sauce

Ingredients

¼ cup extra virgin olive oil
3 cloves of garlic, minced
1 onion, finely chopped (about 1 cup)
1 carrot, peeled and grated
2 (28 oz.) cans of crushed tomatoes
11/2 cup water (for richer flavor try half water and half red wine)
2 Tablespoons fresh oregano, minced (or one teaspoon dried)

1 ½ teaspoons dried fennel seed
2 Tablespoons chopped fresh parsley
1 teaspoon salt
pepper to taste
1 teaspoon red chili pepper flakes
fresh chopped basil and grated Parmesan cheese for topping (optional)

Directions

Place your oil to get hot in a Dutch oven. Sauté the garlic, onion, and carrot until onion is translucent. Toss in all your remaining ingredients and bring to a boil. Switch the heat to low, cover then allow to simmer for about 30 minutes. **N.B** This basic recipe can be easily modified by adding ground beef or turkey, meatballs, mushrooms, or anything that strikes your fancy. Pour it over cooked spaghetti squash (or whole grain pasta once you've finished the detox), or use it for eggplant and goat cheese lasagna or chicken parmesan.

Serves: 16   Prep Time: 15 mins.   Cooking Time: 30 mins.
Calories: 49   Protein: 2.1g   Carbs: 1.1g   Fat: 2g

Is your belly happy yet?

We sincerely hope that you're pleased with the recipes so far. If not, feel free to send us an email at info@limitlessrecipes.com and tell us what we can improve. We get back to every person who reaches out.

If you are enjoying the recipes then you will love the box set below with over 600 delicious and easy to make recipes.

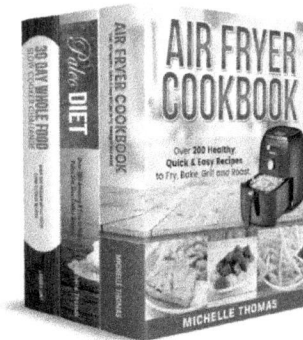

Only sign up for the cookbook box set if you are ready to be absolutely amazed with over 600 proven, delicious and easy to make recipes.

To access the gift page type in www.bit.ly/2Ho82AH or email us at info@limitlessrecipes.com to get the box set delivered to your email.

 Limitless Recipes
Like us on Facebook and join our private Facebook group community for more recipes and gifts.
 @limitlessrecipes
Follow us on Instagram
 Limitless Recipes
Follow us on Pinterest.

Want to be a part of our closed Facebook group?
We are working on building an engaged community discussing recipes and healthy eating in our closed Facebook group. If you would like to be involved in the discussions about cooking, what is working, what is not working and receive information about gifts and promotions, we would be delighted to add you.

Type in Limitless Recipes on Facebook or write us at info@limitlessrecipes.com. Come say hi!

Happy Cooking!

Can we ask you for a quick favor?

We try to write the best cookbooks that we can and a lot of effort goes into writing the cookbook with so many recipes while making sure that the recipes are healthy and fairly easy to make. We sincerely hope you are enjoying the recipes. That being said, reviews really help us A LOT when it comes to putting our names out there and keep us motivated. Competing with big publishing companies is quite hard and reviews really help with making our books more visible.
If you could take one minute to leave a review, we would really appreciate that.

You can leave a review in 3 easy steps:
1. Go to the product page
2. Scroll down and on the left side click 'Write customer review'
3. Write a review and click 'Submit'

Thank you so much. **You are amazing!**

If you feel like we could improve the cookbook please email us at info@limitlessrecipes.com and we'll make sure to get back to you.

Feel free to proceed to the snacks, side dish & spread recipes, yummy!

PREDIABETES DIET SNACKS, SIDE DISH & SPREAD RECIPES

28. Savory Stuffed Mushrooms

Ingredients

24 small/medium mushrooms
1 Tablespoon olive oil
½ cup finely chopped carrots
¼ cup finely chopped celery
¼ cup finely chopped yellow onion

2 cloves minced garlic
½ pound ground beef
2 finely chopped teaspoons rosemary
1 teaspoon sea salt
1 teaspoon black pepper

Directions

Preheat oven to 375° F. Line a baking sheet with aluminum foil. Wipe the mushrooms with a damp kitchen towel or paper towel and remove the stems. Using a spoon, remove the gills from the underside of the mushroom cap. Set prepared mushrooms aside. With stove set to medium, heat olive oil and add carrots, garlic, onions, and celery, and cook until just starting to get tender. Add ground beef, and combine and cook with sautéed vegetables. Continue to cook on medium high until the meat is nicely browned. Add the rosemary and stir. Drain off any fat. Stuff the mushroom caps with the ground beef mixture, carefully place them on the foil-lined baking sheet, and bake at 375 F for approximately 10 minutes.

Serves: 8	Prep Time: 15 mins.		Cooking Time: 15 mins.
Calories: 27	Protein: 1g	Carbs: 1g	Fat: 2.4g

29. Cannellini Bean, Lemon and Herb Spread

Ingredients:

1, (15 ounce) can cannellini beans, rinsed and drained
basil 2 tbsp., chopped roughly
1 tablespoon fresh Italian flat leaf parsley, roughly chopped

2 tablespoons extra virgin olive oil
2 teaspoons lemon zest
1 tablespoon fresh lemon juice
kosher salt, ¼ tsp.
black pepper to taste

Directions:

Combine ingredients in a food processor. Process 30 seconds or until smooth. Store in the refrigerator until ready to use.

Serves: 8	Prep Time: 20 mins.		Cooking Time: 0 mins.
Calories: 90	Protein: 4g	Carbs: 11g	Fat: 4g

30. Greek Yogurt Lemon Aioli

Ingredients

½ cup plain Greek yogurt
1 tablespoon olive oil based mayonnaise
Juice of half a lemon
½ teaspoon garlic powder

1 teaspoon fresh dill, roughly chopped
⅛ teaspoon kosher salt
⅛ teaspoon freshly ground black pepper

Directions

Whisk all ingredients in a small bowl. Serve immediately or chill up to 2 days. Use as needed.

Serves: 4	Prep Time: 15 mins.	Cooking Time: 0 mins.

Calories: 30   Protein: 3g   Carbs: 2g   Fat: 1.5g

31. Pineapple Mango Salsa

Ingredients

1 cup chopped mango
1 cup chopped pineapple
¼ cup chopped red onion
2 tablespoons fresh lime juice

½ cup finely chopped cilantro
½ cup chopped red pepper
⅓ cup good quality extra virgin olive oil

Directions

In a medium bowl combine oil, pepper, cilantro, lime juice, onion, pineapple and mango. Mix well.

Serves: 4   Prep Time: 15 mins.   Cooking Time: 0 mins.
Calories: 198   Protein: 1g   Carbs: 14g   Fat: 17g

32. Pineapple Chicken Kabobs

Ingredients

5 tablespoons extra virgin olive oil, divided
3 cloves of garlic, minced
2 teaspoons lemon zest
1 tablespoon fresh parsley, chopped
½ teaspoon freshly ground black pepper
1 teaspoon kosher salt, divided
Chicken breast, 1-pound, skinless, boneless, cubed
10-ounce pineapple, cut into 1 to 2-inch pieces

1 bell pepper, cut into 1 to 2-inch pieces
½ red onion, cut into 1 to inch pieces
1 yellow squash or zucchini, cut into 1 to 2-inch pieces
Juice of 1 lemon
1 cup wild rice
4 - 6 metal or wooden skewers

Directions

In a large bowl, whisk half of the olive oil, garlic, lemon zest, parsley, pepper, and ½ teaspoon of salt. Add chicken and mix well. In a small bowl whisk together remaining olive oil, salt, and lemon juice. Set aside. Heat grill on medium-high heat. Thread chicken, pineapple, and vegetables on skewers in a varied pattern. Brush kabobs with lemon juice and olive oil mixture. Add kabobs to grill and cook 8 to 12 minutes or until chicken is cooked throughout or reaches an internal temperature of 165°F. While kabobs are grilling, cook rice according to package directions. Remove kabobs from grill and serve over rice.

Serves: 4   Prep Time: 10 mins.   Cooking Time: 15 mins.
Calories: 400   Protein: 24g   Carbs: 37g   Fat: 17g

33. Cauliflower Crust Pizza

Ingredients

½ cup almond flour
1 tbsp. grated parmesan cheese
½ tsp. dried oregano
3 ½ cups Cauliflower rice
¼ tsp. dried basil
⅓ cup shredded cheddar cheese
¼ tsp. garlic powder
4 ounces shredded mozzarella cheese
¼ tsp. black pepper

¼ tsp. salt, divided
2 eggs
Cooking spray
1 tsp. canola oil
2 cups kale, chopped
⅛ tsp. crushed red pepper
1 cup prepared pizza sauce

Directions

Preheat oven to 450°F. Set a medium cast-iron pan into the oven to get hot. Add cauliflower rice to a microwavable bowl and cook for about 7 minutes. Transfer to paper towels and wrap tightly, press to extract any excess water. Cool for about 10 minutes. Add your eggs, black pepper, some salt, garlic powder, basil, oregano, cheddar cheese, parmesan, almond flour and cauliflower to a large bowl then mix to form a dough.

Take the skillet from the oven and give it a light coating of cooking spray. Press dough into bottom of skillet. Set to bake for about 15 minutes or until crust is golden brown. Remove from oven. While crust is cooking, heat oil in a medium sauté pan over medium heat. Add in your kale and season to taste. Cook while stirring, for about 5 minutes then set aside. Add the sauce on top, leaving about an inch dry at the edges. Top with kale and mozzarella then continue baking for about another 10 minutes. Place to cool down a bit before serving.

Serves: 3　　　　**Prep Time: 10 mins.**　　　　**Cooking Time: 50 mins.**
Calories: 270　　**Protein: 25g**　　**Carbs: 21g**　　**Fat: 20g**

34. Cauliflower Fried "Rice"

Ingredients

7 cups Cauliflower Rice
2 tablespoons canola oil, divided
1 small onion, diced
3 cloves garlic, minced
1 tablespoon minced ginger
1 ½ cups mushrooms, diced
1 zucchini, cut in one inch pieces
(about 1 ½ cups)

1 cup shredded carrots
3 tablespoons low sodium tamari
or soy sauce, divided
½ cup unsalted cashews
1 green onion, diced
3 eggs, lightly beaten
1 teaspoon sesame oil

Directions

Heat one tablespoon of canola oil in a medium skillet over medium-high heat. Add onion, garlic, and ginger. Cook until fragrant, about 2 minutes. Add mushrooms, zucchini, and carrots. Cook, while stirring, until the veggies are cooked. Add 1 tablespoon tamari, cashews, and green onion. Remove from heat and set aside. Add in your oil In a wok on medium heat. Add cauliflower rice. Cook, while stirring, for about 2 minutes. Using a spoon, create a well in the center of the pan. Add egg and scramble, incorporating it into rice. Add sautéed vegetables, remaining tamari, and sesame oil. Cook, while stirring, for about 2 minutes. Serve.

Serves: 4　　**Prep Time: 15 mins.**　　　　**Cooking Time: 15 mins.**
Calories: 320　　**Protein: 14g**　　**Carbs: 27g**　　**Fat: 20g**

35. Broccoli and Tempeh with Garlic Sauce

Ingredients

1 cup cooked brown rice
3 cloves of garlic, minced
1 tablespoon fresh ginger, minced
1 tablespoon chili garlic sauce
2 tablespoons low sodium tamari
or soy sauce
⅓ cup low sodium vegetable broth
¼ cup water

1 tablespoon pure maple syrup
1, (8 ounce) package tempeh
1 large head broccoli, trimmed
into florets
1 cup chopped asparagus
2 teaspoons cornstarch dissolved in
2 tablespoons water

Directions

In a large frying pan or wok combine garlic, ginger, chili garlic sauce, soy sauce, broth, water, and maple syrup. Stir and heat over medium-high heat. Bring to boil and cook 5 minutes. Add tempeh, broccoli, asparagus, and dissolved cornstarch. Cook 10 minutes over medium heat or until vegetables are tender. Remove from heat and serve over brown rice.

Serves: 3	Prep Time: 10 mins.		Cooking Time: 15 mins.
Calories: 290	Protein: 19g	Carbs: 9g	Fat: 5g

36. Roasted Brussels Sprouts Medley

Ingredients:

¼ pound Brussels sprouts, halved
1 fennel bulb, cut into thin wedges (green parts removed)
2 cups cauliflower florets
3 tablespoons extra virgin olive oil, divided

½ teaspoon freshly ground black pepper
¼ teaspoon kosher salt
1 small head of radicchio, cored and cut into thin wedges.

Directions:

Preheat oven to 400°F. Place Brussels sprouts, fennel, and cauliflower on a large baking sheet. Use half of your oil to drizzle then season to taste. Lightly toss vegetables to coat evenly. Roast in oven for 15 minutes. Remove from vegetables from oven. Add radicchio and drizzle with remaining olive oil. Return to oven and roast an additional 15 minutes or until all vegetables begin to caramelize and brown on edges. Serve immediately.

Serves: 4	Prep Time: 10 mins.		Cooking Time: 30 mins.
Calories: 130	Protein: 3g	Carbs: 9g	Fat: 10g

37. Citrus-Glazed Carrots

Ingredients:

baby carrots, 1 lb., chopped
orange zest, 1 tsp.
orange juice, ½ cup

butter, 2 tbsp., unsalted
honey, 1 tbsp.
rosemary, 2 tsp.

Directions:

Add your honey, butter, juice, zest and carrots in a skillet. Close the lid and allow to cook until the carrots are fully cooked (about 10 minutes). Stir on occasion then add in rosemary. Mix and serve.

Serves: 4	Prep Time: 10 mins.		Cooking Time: 10 mins.
Calories: 111	Protein: 2g	Carbs: 18g	Fat: 4

38.   Roasted Garlic Mashed Cauliflower

Ingredients:

1 head of cauliflower,
cut into florets (about 4 cups)
6 cloves of garlic, quartered
1 tablespoon extra-virgin olive oil

¼ teaspoon freshly ground black pepper
⅛ teaspoon kosher salt
1 tablespoon cream cheese
1 tablespoon chives, finely chopped

Directions:

Preheat oven to 350°F. Place a large piece of aluminum foil over baking sheet. Place cauliflower florets and garlic on top of foil. Drizzle with olive oil and season with salt and pepper. Wrap foil around cauliflower completely, making a purse. There should be no openings. Roast in oven for 40 to 50 minutes. Remove from oven and immediately transfer to a medium sized bowl. Add cream cheese. Blend with a handheld immersion blender, or mash with potato masher. Once cream cheese is melted and incorporated throughout, fold in chives. Serve immediately.

Serves: 3	Prep Time: 10 mins.	Cooking Time: 10 mins.
Calories: 110	Protein: 5g	Carbs: 11g	Fat: 7g

39.   Roasted Cauliflower

Ingredients

1-pound cauliflower (about one medium to large head), trimmed and cut into ¼ inch slices
extra virgin olive oil

sea salt to taste
coarse black pepper

Directions

Preheat oven to 375°F. Place cauliflower in a large mixing bowl and drizzle evenly with olive oil. Season with salt and pepper, and toss. Place cauliflower slices evenly on cookie sheet and drizzle with any remaining oil. Bake about 25 – 30 minutes or until tender and caramelized on edges. Turn once midway through baking. Serve warm or let cool to room temperature. Delicious as is, or sprinkled with a good aged vinegar.

Serves: 4	Prep Time: 15 mins.	Cooking Time: 30 mins.
Calories: 35	Protein: 3.2g	Carbs: 4g	Fat: 3.2g

40.   Cauliflower Mashed "Potatoes"

Ingredients

florets from 1 head of cauliflower
3/4 cup water
2 tablespoons butter

2 tablespoons unsweetened non-dairy milk
2 teaspoons sea salt, + more to taste
1/8 teaspoon ground black pepper

Directions

Add the water and cauliflower to a large pot and bring to a boil. Allow the florets to steam, while covered, on medium heat until tender, maybe 15 minutes. Drain and place cooked florets into a large food processor with the chopping blade inserted. Add the butter, milk, sea salt, and black pepper and process until the mixture looks like mashed potatoes. Taste and, if necessary, add more seasoning, butter, or milk to suit your taste.

Serves: 6	Prep Time: 15 mins.	Cooking Time: 15 mins.
Calories: 47	Protein: 1.6g	Carbs: 5.4g	Fat: 3g

41.   Coconut Lime Cauliflower Rice

Ingredients

1 head cauliflower, cut into florets
2 tablespoons extra virgin olive oil
1 yellow onion, diced
3 garlic cloves, minced

1 cup canned organic lite coconut milk, stirred
zest and juice of 1 lime
salt and fresh ground pepper to taste

Directions

Add florets to the bowl of your food processor and pulse until cauliflower looks like grains of rice. If you have a smaller-size food processor, work in small batches at a time so that the cauliflower doesn't turn into a paste. Using a nonstick skillet over medium high heat, sauté onions in heated olive oil for 2 -3 minutes, until translucent. Stir in garlic and riced cauliflower; cook for 1 minute. Add coconut milk and continue to cook for about 10 minutes, or until the liquid is adsorbed. Switch off the heat then add in your juice and zest. Adjust the seasoning then serve.

Serves: 4   Prep Time: 15 mins.   Cooking Time: 5 mins.
Calories: 69.7   Protein: 2.3g   Carbs: 1.4g   Fat: 4.7g

42.   Charred Green Beans with Crushed Almonds

Ingredients

1-pound green beans
1 ½ Tablespoons olive oil for cooking
¼ teaspoon salt, plus a pinch

1 ½ Tablespoons fresh dill, minced
Juice from one lemon
¼ cup roasted almonds, chopped

Directions

Preheat oven to 400°F. Drizzle olive oil over green beans and toss with salt. Spread a single layer of beans on a large cookie sheet. (You may line it with foil for easier cleanup.) Be careful not to overcrowd beans. When oven has reached the proper temperature, place cookie sheet in oven and roast beans for 10 minutes. Stir, flipping as many beans over as possible, then roast for 8 – 10 minutes more, until beans are blistered and charred. Remove from oven and place in serving bowl. Stir in dill and lemon juice, and top with chopped almonds and a dash of sea salt.

Serves: 4   Prep Time: 15 mins.   Cooking Time: 20 mins.
Calories: 80   Protein: 1.7g   Carbs: 7.1g   Fat: 6g

43. Carrot Zucchini Fritters

Ingredients

2 cups grated zucchini
2 cups grated carrots
2/3 cup almond flour
3 large eggs, lightly beaten

½ cup scallions, sliced
Olive oil for cooking
Sea salt and pepper to taste

Directions

Place grated vegetables in a bowl and sprinkle lightly with salt. Set aside and let the moisture come out for 10 minutes. Using a clean dish towel or cheese cloth, press the vegetables to squeeze out as much liquid as possible. Add eggs, scallions, almond flour, and seasonings to carrot/zucchini mixture. Stir until well mixed. Heat olive oil in pan over medium high heat and spoon about 3 tablespoons of mixture per fritter into pan. Press down with the flat side of a spatula to make a disk shape. Cook in hot oil, turning once, until both sides are golden brown. Transfer fritters onto paper towels so it can drain. Serve.

Serves: 4-6	Prep Time: 15 mins.		Cooking Time: 6 mins.
Calories: 134	Protein: 3.2g	Carbs: 7.9g	Fat: 10.4g

44. Omelet with Spinach and Mushrooms

Ingredients

4 eggs, lightly beaten
sea salt and ground pepper to taste
2 Tablespoons extra virgin olive oil

1 cup spinach leaves, coarsely chopped
1 cup cremini mushrooms or mushrooms of your choice, sliced

Directions

Add your milk, pepper, salt and eggs into a bowl then whisk. Heat the olive oil in a medium non-stick skillet and sauté spinach and mushrooms until spinach is wilted and mushrooms are tender. Drain any excess liquid and place out the way for now. Add in ½ of your egg mixture into your skillet. Allow to cook until it begins to get firm then toss in ½ of your mushroom and spinach. Stir to combine then add in the remaining mushroom and spinach. Continue to stir until fully cooked. Enjoy!

Serves: 2	Prep Time: 15 mins.		Cooking Time: 6 mins.
Calories: 297	Protein: 16.1g	Carbs: 6.3g	Fat: 22.8g

45. Cheesy Baked Eggs with Spinach

Ingredients

4 teaspoons olive oil
12 cups fresh spinach
2 teaspoons minced garlic

1 cup shredded low fat mozzarella cheese
6 eggs

Directions

Preheat oven to 350° F. Place half the oil in a large skillet. Add 1 teaspoon of garlic and half the spinach and sauté for 2-3 minutes, until spinach is wilted. Add 1/2 cup of cheese and stir to combine. Spray 6 ramekins with nonstick cooking spray. Transfer your spinach mixture evenly into 3 ramekins. Heat the other 2 tsp. oil in your skillet; add in your garlic and remaining spinach then continue to cook. Separate among 3 more ramekins. Carefully crack one egg into each ramekin on top of the spinach mixture. Bake for 15 minutes. The yolks should be slightly runny. Season with salt and pepper.

Serves: 6	Prep Time: 15 mins.	Cooking Time: 17 mins.

Calories: 240   Protein: 16.9g   Carbs: 3.7g   Fat: 17.6g

46.   Frittata with Sun-Dried Tomato and Feta

Ingredients

olive oil, 2 teaspoons
garlic, 1 clove, minced
diced onion, 1/2 cup
sun-dried tomatoes, 1/2 cup, drained and chopped
2 eggs

1/2 cup egg whites
1/4 cup unsweetened almond milk
1/2 cup crumbled light feta cheese light
2 chopped scallions

Directions

Set your oil to get hot in a skillet on medium heat. Add garlic and onion, and cook until onion is tender and has lost its crunch. Stir in sun dried tomatoes, and heat for 2-3 minutes. Place eggs, egg whites, and milk in a small bowl and whisk together. Pour mixture into the skillet and sprinkle the feta cheese evenly over the top. Reduce heat to low. Continue cooking on stove top until set around the edges and center is slightly runny. Move skillet to oven and broil frittata for 3-5 minutes. The frittata is done when the center is firm.

Serves: 4   Prep Time: 15 mins.   Cooking Time: 8 mins.
Calories: 188   Protein: 14.2g   Carbs: 7.5g   Fat: 11.4g

PREDIABETES DIET MAIN DISH RECIPES

47. Eggplant and Goat Cheese Lasagna

Ingredients

cooking spray
1 large eggplant, sliced into ¼ inch discs

1 recipe homemade marinara sauce or spaghetti sauce
4 11 oz. log of goat cheese, sliced

Directions

Preheat oven to 375°. Spray cooking spray into a 9x13 baking dish. Lay ¼ of the eggplant slices in a single layer in the bottom of the dish. Cover with a layer of marinara sauce, and dot with ¼ of the sliced cheese. Continue layering three more times with goat cheese layer on top. Bake for 45 – 60 minutes, or until cheese is melted and sauce is bubbling. Allow to rest for about 10 minutes before slicing to serve.

Serves: 6 | Prep Time: 15 mins. | | Cooking Time: 1 hr. 10 mins.
Calories: 549 | Protein: 59.1g | Carbs: 8.1g | Fat: 65.9g

48. Tomato, Garlic, and Mozzarella Chicken Breasts

Ingredients

2 large garlic cloves, mashed and minced
2 tablespoons anchovy paste
1/2 cup finely chopped flat-leaf parsley
4 tablespoons olive oil, divided

Chicken breast, 4, skinless. boneless, halved
2 large plum tomatoes, cut into slices
8 ounces of Mozzarella di Buffalo or Whole Milk Mozzarella cut into slices.

Directions

Stir together black pepper, oil, parsley, anchovy paste and garlic. With a sharp knife, slice through the center of the chicken breasts horizontally, but don't cut all the way through. Spread them open like a fan, lay them flat on your work surface, and pat dry with a clean kitchen towel. Spread parsley mixture over the surface of the chicken and fold chicken pieces in half, forming a pouch.
Insert the tomato slices and cheese into the pouch and brush the outside with oil, salt and pepper.

Season the outside of the chicken breasts with 1/4 teaspoon salt and 1/4 teaspoon pepper, then brush with 1/2 tablespoon oil. If you'd like, use skewers to hold the chicken halves together. Add your remaining oil in a large nonstick skillet over medium-high heat until hot. Add chicken and cook about 2-3 minutes per side, or until nicely browned. Lower heat and cover skillet. Continue cooking until chicken is done, about 5 more minutes. Reserve pan juices and serve on the side of the chicken.

Serves: 4 | Prep Time: 15 mins. | | Cooking Time: 11 mins.
Calories: 322 | Protein: 14g | Carbs: 7.9g | Fat: 26.5g

49.   Italian Deviled Chicken with Tomato and Eggplant

Ingredients

1-pound chicken thighs, skinless and boneless
3 Tablespoons extra-virgin olive oil
Fine salt and black pepper to taste
1/4 tsp hot red pepper flakes to taste
2 small globe eggplants (could also use zucchinis), chopped in 1-inch chunks
1 yellow onion, sliced
2 garlic cloves, sliced

2 large tomatoes, cubed or 1 cup canned plum tomatoes, chopped with juice
3/4 cup chicken broth
12 pitted kalamata olives, halved
1 tablespoon capers, rinsed and drained.
Cornstarch slurry made with equal parts water and cornstarch
2 Tablespoons chopped parsley

Directions

Cut chicken thighs (or chicken breasts) into bite-sized pieces that will cook evenly. Heat 2 Tablespoons of olive oil in skillet and brown chicken on both sides. Transfer to plate and season with salt, pepper, and red pepper flakes. Add another 1 Tablespoon of olive oil to the same pan and brown eggplant, onion, and garlic for 5 minutes until soft.

Return chicken to skillet, add tomatoes, and stir. Add chicken broth, bring to a boil and simmer partially covered for 15 minutes. Turn the chicken pieces over and add olives and capers, and cook for an additional 10 minutes or until chicken is cooked through. Stir in corn starch mixture and simmer, stirring, until sauce thickens.

Serves: 4   **Prep Time: 15 mins.**   **Cooking Time: 11 mins.**
Calories: 464   **Protein: 32.2g**   **Carbs: 21.5g**   **Fat: 28.4g**

50. Chicken Thighs Roasted with Lemon and Fennel

Ingredients

6 chicken thighs
2 small fennel bulbs
4 large garlic cloves, minced
zest and juice from 1 lemon

2 tablespoons olive oil
2 tablespoons dry white wine
teaspoon kosher salt
Freshly ground black pepper

Directions

Place oven rack in the center of the oven and preheat to 425°F. Place the chicken thighs in a large bowl; set aside. Cut the fronds and the ends of the stalks off the fennel bulbs, setting fronds aside. Slice each bulb into quarters and then slice into 1-inch-thick segments. Chop about 1 tablespoon of the fennel fronds and add to the chicken along with fennel slices. Add garlic, lemon zest, lemon juice, oil, and white wine. Season with salt and pepper and toss ingredients until well combined.

Arrange the mixture on a large cooking sheet covered with foil. The fennel should be placed around the outside of the sheet and the chicken pieces should be close together in the center. Any juices remaining in the bowl can be poured over the chicken. Roast in preheated oven about 30 minutes, until the chicken is brown and crispy and no pink juices are running out. Internal temperature should be about 160°F. The fennel should be tender and slightly brown around the edges. Remove the pan from the oven and cover with another sheet of aluminum foil. Let sit for approximately 5 to 10 minutes, and serve.

Serves: 4	**Prep Time: 15 mins.**	**Cooking Time: 30 mins.**
Calories: 764	**Protein: 49.9g**	**Carbs: 15.8g**	**Fat: 55.2g**

51. Ground Turkey with Quinoa, Kale, Tomatoes, and Mushrooms

Ingredients

1 tablespoon olive oil
1-pound lean ground turkey
one small yellow onion, thinly sliced, then halved
salt and pepper to taste
1-pound mushrooms, sliced
4 cups baby kale leaves, tightly packed
2 cups chopped tomatoes (or use canned tomatoes)

3/4 cup dry white wine
3 cups cooked quinoa
1 Tablespoon fresh parsley, chopped
1 ½ teaspoons fresh oregano, chopped
1 ½ teaspoon fresh basil, chopped
Parmesan cheese

Directions

Set your oil to get hot in a skillet on high heat. Add onions and cook until translucent. Add turkey, salt, and pepper. Start breaking the turkey up into pieces then cook until turkey is cooked through and brown. Remove turkey mixture from pan and set aside. Add mushrooms to pan, working in small batches if necessary. Sauté until golden brown. Add kale and tomatoes to mushrooms and continue cooking until the kale is cooked. Turn the heat up to high then add turkey and onion mixture. Add wine and allow to boil. Switch the heat to low and allow the wine to simmer until it has reduced by half. Stir in quinoa and herbs and continue cooking until warmed through. Top with a dash of parmesan cheese and serve.

Serves: 4	**Prep Time: 20 mins.**	**Cooking Time: 30 mins.**
Calories: 478	**Protein: 37g**	**Carbs: 39.4g**	**Fat: 20.7g**

52. Slow and Easy Pork Chops

Ingredients

½ cup plus ¼ cup all-purpose flour
½ teaspoon ground mustard
½ teaspoon garlic pepper
¼ teaspoon seasoned salt

4 - 4 oz. boneless loin pork chops
2 Tablespoons olive oil
1 ½ cups homemade chicken broth

Directions

Place ½ cup flour, ground mustard, and seasonings in a large resealable plastic bag and shake until combined. Add each pork chop to bag, one at a time, and shake bag until pork chop is coated. Set your oil to heat in a skillet on medium heat. Quickly brown pork chops on both sides. Move pork chops to a large (5 qt.) slow cooker. Take remaining ¼ cup flour and whisk in chicken broth until smooth. Pour mixture into slow cooker to cover pork chops. Cover, cook on low setting for 3-4 hours. Remove meat to a serving dish and transfer cooking liquid to a mixing bowl. Whisk until you have a smooth sauce, serve on the side, or pour over pork chops.

Serves: 4	Prep Time: 15 mins.	Cooking Time: 30 mins.
Calories: 764	Protein: 49.9g	Carbs: 15.8g	Fat: 55.2g

53. Spicy Pork Pot Roast

Ingredients:

2 medium dried ancho chilis, stem and seeds removed
3 medium dried guajillo chilis, stem and seeds removed
2 bay leaves
2 Tablespoons cider vinegar
1 small yellow or white onion, coarsely chopped
3 cloves garlic, chopped

1 tsp thyme, marjoram or oregano (ideally a mix of all three)
1/4 tsp fresh ground allspice
1/4 tsp fresh ground cloves
1 1/2 Tablespoons vegetable oil
1/2 tsp Kosher salt
3 1/2 lbs. boneless pork shoulder or butt roast, or bone-in pork shoulder roast with some skin left on

Directions

Place the chilis in a small bowl, fill with hot water and let stand for 10-20 minutes to rehydrate. Put a heavy cup on top of the chilis to keep them submerged. Transfer the chilis plus a cup of liquid to the blender. Grind the spices in a spice grinder, then add to the blender along with the vinegar, onion, garlic, and mixed herbs. Process to a smooth puree.

With a boneless cut, slice into 3 inches thick slabs. Place the roast in a large roasting pot and spoon or rub the chili paste all over, working into the incisions. Pour the remaining cup of water around the meat, cover, bring to a boil, and simmer for about 2 1/2 hours. Let the pork stand, covered, for about 20 minutes before serving. The meat should be fork tender. Remove the bone, shred, and serve.

Serves: 8	Prep Time: 20 mins.	Cooking Time: 2 hrs. 30 mins.
Calories: 302	Protein: 44.6g	Carbs: 1.3g	Fat: 11.8g

54. Easy Fisherman's Stew

Ingredients

6 Tablespoons olive oil

3 large garlic cloves, minced

1 ½ cups chopped onion (about one medium onion)

2/3 cup fresh chopped parsley

1 ½ cups chopped tomato (or use a 14-ounce can of tomatoes, whole or crushed, with their juices)

2 teaspoons tomato paste (optional)

8 oz. of clam juice

½ cup dry white wine

1 ½ lb. firm white fish fillets, cut into 2-inch pieces (good choices are halibut, cod, red snapper, or sea bass)

Pinch of dried oregano

Pinch of dried thyme

1/8 teaspoon Tabasco sauce (or to taste)

Salt and freshly ground black pepper to taste

Directions

In a large heavy pot over medium-high heat, heat olive oil, and add onion. Sauté for about 4 minutes, then add the minced garlic and cook an additional minute. Add parsley, stir for 2 minutes. Stir in tomatoes and tomato paste, and allow to simmer gently for about 10 minutes. Pour in dry white wine and clam juice, then add fish pieces. Return to simmering for about 3 to 5 minutes, until the fish is cooked through and flakes apart easily. Add spices and Tabasco, and salt to taste. Serve in bowls.

Serves: 4	Prep Time: 20 mins.		Cooking Time: 2 hrs. 30 mins.
Calories: 302	Protein: 44.6g	Carbs: 1.3g	Fat: 11.8g

55. Easy grilled salmon

Ingredients

1 pound wild-caught salmon filet, rinsed, dried, quartered

1 teaspoon dried basil

1 teaspoon dried oregano

1 teaspoon black pepper

1 teaspoon salt

1/4 cup extra virgin olive oil

2 cloves minced garlic

Juice of 1 lemon

Directions

Combine pepper, salt, oregano, basil, garlic, lemon juice and olive oil in a jar, place the lid on tightly and shake well to mix. Pour on top of your salmon, set in a baking dish then turn it over to fully coat. Place in the refrigerator to marinate 1 hour before grilling. Preheat grill to medium-high. Grill salmon 4 minutes on each side. Enjoy!

Serves: 4	Prep Time: 20 mins.		Cooking Time: 8 mins.
Calories: 465	Protein: 17g	Carbs: 86.9g	Fat: 7.1g

56. Mustard Braised Short Ribs

Ingredients

2 pounds boneless beef short ribs
1 tablespoon olive oil
sea salt and pepper
4 cloves of garlic, mashed
3 cups natural beef broth

1 cup Dijon mustard
3/4 cup of your favorite unsweetened non-dairy milk
1/4 teaspoon sea salt
8-10 sprigs of fresh thyme

Directions

Preheat the oven to 325°F. Before braising, allow short ribs to come to room temperature. Dry with paper towels and sprinkle all sides generously with sea salt and freshly ground black pepper. Heat olive oil over medium-high heat in a large oven-proof Dutch oven. Add the short ribs to the pan and cook for 3-5 minutes without turning, so that a dark crust forms on one side. Do the same on all sides of the ribs. The garlic cloves can be cooked alongside the short ribs, until both sides are a golden brown. Transfer to a plate.

Deglaze the pot by adding the beef broth and stirring with a wooden spoon, making sure to scrape up the bits at the bottom of the pan. Whisk in the thyme, salt, milk and mustard until evenly combined. Allow the flavors to blend by bringing mixture to a simmer for 3 minutes. Return the short ribs and garlic to the Dutch oven and cover with a lid. Place in preheated oven, for 2 1/2 hours. Serve with a side of mashed or roasted cauliflower.

Serves: 4-6   **Prep Time: 20 mins.**   **Cooking Time: 8 mins.**
Calories: 580   **Protein: 32.9g**   **Carbs: 14.2g**   **Fat: 44.6g**

57.   Onion and Peas Soup

Ingredients:

Peas (1 cup, boiled)
Carrots (2, peeled, chopped)
Onion (1, sliced)
Chicken broth (2 cups)
Lemon juice (1 tablespoon)

Garlic (4-5 cloves, minced)
Black pepper (½ teaspoon)
Salt (¼ teaspoon)
Oil (1 tablespoon)

Directions:

Heat oil in a saucepan, add onion and garlic cloves, fry for 2 minutes. Add all peas and carrots stir for 5 minutes. Add chicken broth, salt, pepper, and mix well. Allow to cook for about 15 minutes on low heat. Strain and ladle into serving bowls. Drizzle lemon juice. Serve and enjoy.

Serves: 3	**Prep Time: 15 mins.**	**Cook Time: 25 mins.**
Calories: 115	**Protein: 7g** **Carbs: 21g**	**Fat: 0g**

58.   Curried Carrot, Sweet Potato, and Ginger Soup

Ingredients:

Extra Virgin Olive Oil (2 tsp.)
Shallots (½ cup, chopped)

Sweet Potato (3 cups, peeled, cubed)
Carrots (1½ cup, peeled, sliced)

Directions:

Place a saucepan with your oil on medium heat until it just begins to smoke. Add your shallots to the pot and sauté until it becomes tender (should take approximately 2 – 3 min). Add all your prepped vegetables to the shallots, and your curry then allow to cook for another 2 minutes. Pour in your broth and allow it to come to a boil. Once boiling, place the lid on the pot and reduce the heat to low. Allow this mixture to simmer until your vegetables are all tender. Once tender, add salt and pour your soup into a food processor. Pulse until creamy and smooth. Strain, serve and Enjoy. Tip: Consider topping with a teaspoon of vanilla Greek yogurt and sesame seeds.

Serves: 3	**Prep Time: 10 mins.**	**Cook Time: 25 mins.**
Calories: 144	**Protein: 4.1g** **Carbs: 27.3g**	**Fat: 2.3g**

59. Creamy Cauliflower Soup

Ingredients:

cauliflower (14oz., cut into florets)
watercress (5oz.)
spinach (7oz., thawed)
chicken stock (8 cups)

ghee (¼ cup)
Salt and pepper (1 tsp. each to taste)
Onion (1, chopped)
Garlic (2 cloves, crushed)

Directions:

Grease Dutch oven with ghee, place over medium-high heat and add onion and garlic. Cook until browned and stir cauliflower florets. Cook for 5 minutes. Add spinach and water cress and cook for 2 minutes or until just wilted, pour in vegetable stock and bring to boil. Cook until cauliflower is crisp-tender and stir in the coconut milk. Season to taste then switch off the heat. Allow cooling and puree the soup in Blender until creamy. Strain and serve immediately.

Serves: 6   **Prep Time: 15 mins.**   **Cook Time: 15 mins.**
Calories: 105   **Protein: 4g**   **Carbs: 6g**   **Fat: 8g**

60. Cream of Corn Soup

Ingredients:

Corn puree (0.5 lb.)
Carrots (0.5 lb., cut into ½-inch pieces)
vegetable stock (2 cups)
onion (½ cup, chopped)
salt (½ teaspoon)

Pepper (¼ teaspoon)
Thyme (1 teaspoon, dried)
celery (2 oz., chopped)
olive oil (½ tablespoon)
anise star (1)

Directions:

Heat olive oil in medium pot and add onion; add celery, carrots and sauté for 15 minutes, until onion is caramelized. Add in corn and stir until corn is tender. Add thyme and stir well. Transfer the vegetables in a Blender, add pumpkin puree, vegetable stock, and pulse until smooth. Transfer the mixture into sauce pan and simmer, add anise star and simmer over medium-high heat for 5-8 minutes or until heated through. Remove the anise star and discard. Serve immediately.

Serves: 4   **Prep Time: 10 mins.**   **Cook Time: 25 mins.**
Calories: 294   **Protein: 12.9g**   **Carbs: 56g**   **Fat: 8.3g**

61. Chestnut Soup

Ingredients:

Chestnuts (30oz., whole, roasted)
Shallot (1, roughly chopped)
bacon (3 slices, chopped)
heavy cream (½ cup)
chicken stock (½ cup)
leek (1, white and light green parts chopped)

butter (2 tablespoons)
thyme (1 sprig)
bay leaf (1)
celery (1 stalk, chopped)
nutmeg (½ teaspoon)
Salt and pepper, to taste

Directions:

Cook bacon in an in a medium saucepot for 3-4 minutes. Add butter, carrot, leek, shallot, and celery. Allow to cook until vegetables were cooked (about 6 minutes). Add stock, thyme, bay leaf, chestnuts and bring to boil. Reduce heat and simmer for 25 minutes. Remove from the heat and discard the thyme and bay leaf. Allow to cool slightly and puree using an immersion blender. Reheat the soup and stir in the cream, nutmeg and season to taste. Cook for 5 minutes more. Serve while still hot.

Serves: 6-7   **Prep Time: 10 mins.**   **Cook Time: 50 mins.**
Calories: 280   **Protein: 6g**   **Carbs: 25g**   **Fat: 18g**

62. Coconut Mushroom Soup

Ingredients:

Mushrooms (1 cup, sliced)
coconut milk (1 cup)
onion (1, sliced)
chicken broth (1 cup)

garlic (4-5 cloves, minced)
black pepper (½ teaspoon)
salt (¼ teaspoon)
oil (1 tablespoon)

Directions:

Heat oil in a saucepan, add onion and garlic cloves, cook for 1 minute. Add all mushroom and fry for 5 minutes. Add chicken broth, coconut milk, salt, pepper and mix well. Allow to cook for about 15 minutes on low heat. Transfer to serving bowls. Serve and enjoy.

Serves: 3   **Prep Time: 10 mins.**   **Cook Time: 50 mins.**
Calories: 180   **Protein: 3g**   **Carbs: 7g**   **Fat: 2g**

63. Split pea & Quinoa Soup

Ingredients:

split peas (1 cup, yellow)

Quinoa (½ cup, uncooked)

vegetable broth (4 cups)

bay leaf (½)

coriander seeds (¼ teaspoon, ground)

olive oil (½ tablespoon)

Salt and pepper, to taste

Directions:

Rinse the peas under cold water and remove any black ones. Place the rinsed peas into a saucepan. Add your remaining ingredients to the pot and stir. Cover and cook for 60 minutes. Season to taste and serve while still hot.

Serves: 4   **Prep Time: 10 mins.**   **Cook Time: 1 hr.**

Calories: 224   **Protein: 13.7g**   **Carbs: 41.8g**   **Fat: 0g**

64. Quinoa and Vegetable soup

Ingredients:

Tomatoes (8oz. can, fire roasted)

Carrots (2, diced)

vegetable broth (6 cups)

coriander seeds (¼ teaspoon, ground)

olive oil (1 tablespoon)

Quinoa (8oz., uncooked)

celery (2 stalks, chopped)

cumin (¼ teaspoon, ground)

Salt and pepper, to taste

Directions:

Place all ingredients into a cooker. Stir and set the cooker to simmer. Cook for 45 minutes. Season to taste before serving.

Serves: 8   **Prep Time: 10 mins.**   **Cook Time: 50 mins.**

Calories: 114   **Protein: 15g**   **Carbs: 8g**   **Fat: 2g**

65. Pureed Chicken Noodles with Chicken Thighs

Ingredients

Fresh noodles (24 oz.)
Garlic (6 cloves, minced)
Oil (3 Tablespoons)
Chicken Broth (4 ½ cups)
Water (1 ½ cups)
Mushrooms- Shiitake (12, sliced)

Carrots (12 slices)
Baby bok choy (12)
White Pepper (1/4 teaspoon)
Salt (1/4 teaspoon)
Chicken Thighs (12 oz., skinless, boneless, cooked, and shredded)

Directions

Boil noodles till al dente, then rinse and drain. Put aside till needed. Stir fry garlic in oil till golden, put aside. Heat broth and water then add carrot, mushrooms, bok choy, salt, and pepper to taste. When veggies have cooked, remove from heat. Add chicken noodles and chicken thighs in a food processor and process until you have achieved an apple sauce consistency. Serve and top with a dash of garlic oil on top to finish.

Serves: 3　　　　**Prep Time: 10 mins.**　　　**Cook Time: 20 mins.**
Calories: 375　　　**Protein: 22.5g**　　　**Carbs: 36.7g**　　　**Fat: 16.3g**

66. Smashed Potato Salad

Ingredients

Potatoes (3lbs, Yukon gold, quartered, boiled and mashed)
Eggs (4 hard boiled, sliced)
Celery (1 stalk, chopped)
Radishes (6, thinly sliced)

Sweet Pickle Relish (2 tbsp.)
Green Onions (3, thinly sliced)
Miracle Whip Dressing (3/4 cup)
Vinegar (1 tbsp., white)
Paprika (1/2 tsp.)

Directions:

Add your warm potatoes to a bowl with all your remaining ingredients and mix to fully combine. Serve and enjoy.

Serves: 6　　　　**Prep Time: 10 mins.**　　　**Cook Time: 35 mins.**
Calories: 204　　　**Protein: 5g**　　　**Carbs: 25g**　　　**Fat: 9g**

67. Pureed Roasted Sweet Potato Salad

Ingredients

Sweet Potatoes (2lbs, chopped and roasted)
Onion (¼ cup, chopped)
Green Bell Peppers (1, seeded, and chopped)
Mixed Vegetable (1 can drained)
Salt and Pepper (to taste)

Eggs (3, hard – boiled, chopped)
Dill (1 tbsp., chopped)
Mayonnaise (½ Cup)
Yellow Mustard (1 tsp.)

Directions:

Add your warm potatoes to a bowl with all your remaining ingredients and mix to fully combine. Add to a food processor and pulse until completely pureed. Serve warm or chilled.

Serves: 6   **Prep Time: 20 mins.**   **Cook Time: 45 mins.**
Calories: 177   **Protein: 7.5g**   **Carbs: 37.4g**   **Fat: 1g**

68. Pureed Kale Curry

Ingredients

kale leaves (2 cups, chopped)
chicken broth (2 cups)
garlic paste (1 teaspoon)
ginger (2-inch, sliced, shredded)
turmeric powder (¼ teaspoon)

salt (¼ teaspoon)
chili (1 green)
coconut oil (1 tablespoon)
water (½ cup)

Directions

In a blender add kale with water and green chili, blend till puree. Now heat oil in a pan and add ginger with garlic, sauté for 1 minute. Add kale and fry for 5 minutes or its color is slightly changed. Pour chicken broth and add salt, leave to cook on low heat for 15-20 minutes. Serve and enjoy.

Serves: 5   **Prep Time: 10 mins.**   **Cook Time: 30 mins.**
Calories: 269.5   **Protein: 7.9g**   **Carbs: 48.5g**   **Fat: 6.3g**

69. Baked Chicken Parmesan

Ingredients

chicken breast, 32 oz., trimmed and halved
breadcrumbs, ¾ cup, seasoned
Parmesan Cheese, ¼ cup, grated
butter, 2 tbsp., melted

mozzarella cheese, ¾ cup, shredded
tomato sauce (8 tbsp.)
cooking spray

Directions

Set your oven to preheat to 450 degrees and use your spray to lightly grease your baking sheet. Mix together your parmesan and breadcrumbs in a bowl. Use your butter to lightly brush the chicken then dip into the breadcrumb mixture. Transfer to the baking sheet. Give each piece of chicken another light coating of oil then set to bake for about 20 minutes in the oven. Turn chicken over bake another 5 minutes. Glaze with a tbsp sauce over each piece of chicken then add a dash of mozzarella cheese. Set to bake for another 5 minutes so that the cheese melts..

Serves: 8   **Prep Time: 10 mins.**   **Cook Time: 30 mins.**
Calories: 251   **Protein: 31.5g**   **Carbs: 14g**   **Fat: 9.5g**

70. Thai Green Curry Chicken

Ingredients

1 ½ Cans Light Coconut Milk
3 Tbsp. Green Curry Paste
4 Garlic Cloves
3 Tbsp. Brown Sugar
2 ½ lbs. Chicken Breast, Cut Into Chunks

1 Bag Stir Fry Vegetables
1 Red Onions
1 Can Mini Corn
2 Tbsp. Cornstarch

Directions

Whisk together the coconut milk, curry paste, garlic cloves, and brown sugar. Add the chicken, baby corn, onion, and vegetables. Then cook for four hours on low. After the cooking is finished, whisk together the cornstarch and add 2 tablespoons of water. Cook everything for another thirty minutes or until the curry is thickened.

Serves: 1   **Prep Time: 15 mins.**   **Cook Time: 4 hrs. 30 mins.**
Calories: 298   **Protein: 35.5g**   **Carbs: 5.9g**   **Fat: 10.5g**

71. Turkey Herb Roast

Ingredients

½ Cup Cream Cheese
1/ 3 tsp. Garlic Powder
1/ 3 tsp. Dried Thyme
3 lbs. Turkey Breast
2 ½ Tbsp. Butter

1 Tbsp. Parsley
1 1/ 3 Tbsp. Soy Sauce
½ tsp. Sage
½ tsp. Basil
½ tsp. Pepper

Directions

Mix all the ingredients together in a bowl and brush it over the turkey breast. Place the breast and remaining ingredients in the slow cooker and cook for ten hours on low or six hours on high.

Serves: 2   **Prep Time: 5 mins.**   **Cook Time: 6 hrs.**
Calories: 468   **Protein: 77.1g**   **Carbs: 2.1g**   **Fat: 41g**

72. Turkey Mercedes

Ingredients:

3 Garlic Cloves
Pepper, 1 Tbsp.
Cumin, 1 Tbsp.
Oregano, 1 Tbsp.
Salt, 2 Tbsp.

Lemon Juice, 2 C.
White Wine, 1 C.
Orange Juice, ½ Can, frozen
Turkey, 16 lbs.

Directions

Place turkey in the crockpot and mix ingredients together in a food process to blend gently. Put everything in the crockpot and cook on high for eight hours. Check for doneness.

Serves: 1   **Prep Time: 15 mins.**   **Cook Time: 8 hrs.**
Calories: 634   **Protein: 74.5g**   **Carbs: 8.9g**   **Fat: 25.6g**

73. Navy Style Turkey

Ingredients

1 (18lb.) Turkey
1 ¼ C. Butter
1 lb. Baby Carrots
2 Onions
3 Stalks Celery
1 Garlic Clove

3 Tbsp. Thyme
3 Tbsp. Sage
2 Bay Leaves
1 Bottle Chardonnay Salt and Pepper

Directions

Remove the neck and giblet from the turkey and rinse the bird, then pat it dry. Place it in the crockpot and put the butter under the turkey's skin and secure it with toothpicks. Then mix together the onions, carrots, celery, garlic cloves, sage, thyme, bay leaves, salt, and pepper. Stuff the turkey with as much of this as possible. Pour the bottle of Chardonnay over the bird and roast for 8 hours on high.

Serves: 1   **Prep Time: 15 mins.**   **Cook Time: 8 hrs.**
Calories: 786   **Protein: 111.3g**   **Carbs: 7.3g**   **Fat: 53.7g**

74. Flavorful Turkey Cook

Ingredients

½ C. Butter
1 (12 lb.) Turkey
1 Tbsp. Olive Oil
2 Apples
1 Onion

½ Garlic head
1 lb. Celery
1 Tbsp. Poultry Seasoning

Directions

Rub the skin of the bird with the olive oil and stuff it with the remaining ingredients, except the butter. Place the butter under the skin and cook on high for eight hours, or until the bird reads 180 ° F.

Serves: 1   **Prep Time: 15 mins.**   **Cook Time: 8 hrs.**
Calories: 556   **Protein: 91.3g**   **Carbs: 6.1g**   **Fat: 40.3g**

75.   Three Bean Turkey Chili

Ingredients

1.3 lb. fat free ground turkey breast

1 small onion chopped

1 can of diced tomatoes

1 can of tomato sauce

1 can chopped chilies drained

1 can of chickpeas undrained

1 can of black beans undrained

1 can of small red beans undrained

2 tbsp of chili powder

For Topping:

½ cup of red chopped onion ½ cup of fresh cilantro shredded cheddar

Directions

Brown turkey and onion over a medium high heat in a skillet until cooked through. Drain any excess fat from it and transfer to slow cooker. Add chili powder, tomato sauce, tomatoes, chickpeas, chilies and beans then mix well. Add in your slow cooker and allow to cook for 8 hours on high.

Serves: 12   **Prep Time: 15 mins.**   **Cook Time: 6-8 hrs.**

Calories: 206.3   **Protein: 16.8g**   **Carbs: 31.8g**   **Fat: 40.3g**

76.   Simple Beef Pot Roast

Ingredients

1 5 lb. Beef Pot Roast Salt and Pepper

1 Tbsp. Flour

2 Tbsp. Olive Oil

8 Ounces Mushrooms, sliced

1 Onion

2 Garlic Cloves, minced

1 Tbsp. Butter

1 ½ Tbsp. Flour

1 Tbsp. Tomato Paste

2 ½ C. Chicken Broth

3 Carrots

2 Celery Stalks

1 Sprig Rosemary

2 Sprigs Thyme

Directions

Rinse and pat dry the roast and sprinkle with salt and pepper. Sprinkle the flour over the roast until it's well coated and shake off any excess. Heat the vegetables in a skillet until they're hot, and then sear the roast on both sides for five to six minutes until it's well browned. Transfer from the skillet and set aside.

Add the onion, garlic, and mushrooms and cook for five minutes with each addition. Then add 1 ½ Tbsp. flour and cook for another minute. Add in your tomato paste and leave to cook for a minute. Pour in your stock and stir. Place the carrots and celery in the slow cooker. Put the roast over the vegetables and add the rosemary and thyme. Then add the onion and mushroom and cover the slow cooker. Cook on high for five to six hours.

Serves: 2   **Prep Time: 20 mins.**   **Cook Time: 6 hrs. 30 mins.**

Calories: 368   **Protein: 54.5g**   **Carbs: 7.5g**   **Fat: 57.3g**

77.   Mexican Style Meat

Ingredients

1 (4 lb.) Chuck Roast
1 tsp. Salt
1 tsp. Pepper
2 Tbsp. Olive Oil
1 Onion

1 ¼ C. Green Chile Pepper, diced
1 tsp. Chili Powder
1 tsp. Ground Cayenne
1 5oz. Bottle Hot Pepper Sauce
1 tsp. Garlic Powder

Directions

Trim the roast of excess fat and season with salt and pepper. Heat the olive oil in a skillet and sear the beef. Transfer the roast to the slow cooker and top it with chopped onion. Season the roast with the rest of the ingredients and cook on high for six hours. Then reduce it to low and cook for another two to four hours.

Serves: 2   **Prep Time: 30 mins.**   **Cook Time: 8 hrs.**
Calories: 235   **Protein: 18.4g**   **Carbs: 3.3g**   **Fat: 19.1g**

78.   Beef Pot Roast II

Ingredients

Cream of Mushroom Soup, 21.5 oz. canned, Condensed
Dry Onion Soup Mix, 1oz.

Water, 1 ¼ C.
Roast, 5 ½ lb.

Directions

Mix the water, soup mix, and mushroom soup in the crockpot. Then place the roast in and coat with the soup mixture. Cook on high for three to four hours and low for eight to nine hours.

Serves: 2   **Prep Time: 15 mins.**   **Cook Time: 11 hrs.**
Calories: 465   **Protein: 45.6g**   **Carbs: 4.9g**   **Fat: 23.7g**

79.   Roast Beef

Ingredients

3 lb. Rump Roast
Cream of Mushroom Soup, 21.5 oz. canned, Condensed

Beef Broth, 10.75 oz., canned, condensed

Directions

Place all ingredients in the slow cooker and cook for eight hours on low.

Serves: 2   **Prep Time: 15 mins.**   **Cook Time: 8 hrs.**
Calories: 348   **Protein: 35.3g**   **Carbs: 3.3g**   **Fat: 16.1g**

80. Asian Style Ribs

Ingredients

¼ C. Brown Sugar

1 C. Soy Sauce

¼ C. Sesame Oil

2 Tbsp. Olive Oil

2 Tbsp. Rice Vinegar

2 Tbsp. Lime Juice

2 Tbsp. Minced Garlic

2 Tbsp. Ginger

1 tsp. Sriracha Hot Pepper Sauce

12 Pork Ribs

Directions

Stir together the brown sugar up to the Sriracha sauce and place it in the crock pot. Then add the ribs, cover and refrigerate for at least eight hours or overnight. Then drain the marinade and discard. Cook for nine hours on low. Drain the meat and shred it using two forks.

Serves: 2   **Prep Time: 10 mins.**   **Cook Time: 17 hrs.**

Calories: 526   **Protein: 48.4g**   **Carbs: 13.9g**   **Fat: 44g**

81. Spicy Green Chili Pork

Ingredients

1 Onion Salt and Pepper

2 ½ Lb. Pork Shoulder Roast

1 16 oz. Jar Green Salsa

½ C. Chopped Cilantro, Fresh

2 Serrano Chile Peppers

Directions

Layer the onions in the bottom of the slow cooker and season the pork shoulder with salt and pepper. Place the pork shoulder on top of the onions and pour the green salsa over top. Sprinkle the cilantro over the pork and add in your peppers.

Continue to cook until the meat is fully cooked, about eight hours. Transfer the pork to a cutting board then toss out the liquid from the pot. Then discard the onions and peppers. Shred the pork and mix it with the reserved liquid before serving.

Serves: 2   **Prep Time: 10 mins.**   **Cook Time: 8 hrs.**

Calories: 215   **Protein: 15.9g**   **Carbs: 5.4g**   **Fat: 8.4g**

82. Lancaster County Pork and Sauerkraut

Ingredients:

1 4lb. Pork Loin Roast

1 tsp. Caraway Seeds Salt and Pepper

2 C. Sauerkraut

Directions

Cut the loin if you need to in order to fit it into the slow cooker. Season it with the caraway seeds, salt and pepper to your taste. Add your sauerkraut on your roast then set to cook for 1 hour on high. Switch to low heat and continue to cook for about 6 hours.

Serves: 2   **Prep Time: 20 mins.**   **Cook Time: 6 hrs.**

Calories: 392   **Protein: 36.8g**   **Carbs: 3.5g**   **Fat: 8.5g**

83. Pork Roast with Sauerkraut and Kielbasa

Ingredients:

1 2lb. Pork Loin Roast, Boneless
2 Tbsp. Olive Oil
2 Sprigs Thyme Leaves Salt and Pepper

4 lbs. Sauerkraut
1 lb. Kielbasa, cut in 3 in. pieces

Directions

Preheat your broiler and place the roast on a roasting pan. Then brush the roast with olive oil, sprinkle it with the thyme leaves, and season it with the salt and pepper. Place it in the broiler for ten minutes or until it's browned in several places. Then put the sauerkraut in the slow cooker and arrange the kielbasa pieces around the edges. Put the roast in the center and cover it with the sauerkraut using a fork. Cook it on high for six hours or until it's tender.

Serves: 2   **Prep Time: 25 mins.**   **Cook Time: 6 hrs.**
Calories: 254   **Protein: 14.8g**   **Carbs: 7.6g**   **Fat: 15.7 g**

84. Oven Fried Breaded Pork Chops

Ingredients

pork chops, 6, boneless, fat trimmed
kosher salt
egg, 1 large, beaten
panko crumbs, ½ cup
cornflakes, 1/ 3 cup, crushed
Parmesan cheese, 2 tbsp., grated

sweet paprika, 1 ¼ tsp.
garlic powder, ½ tsp.
chili powder, ¼ tsp.
onion powder, ½ tsp.
black pepper, 1/ 8 tsp

Directions

Set your oven to preheat to 425 and lightly grease your baking sheet. Season pork chops with salt. Combine pepper, chili powder, onion powder, garlic powder, paprika, salt, parmesan cheese, cornflakes and panko. Place beaten egg in another. Dredge your pork into your eggs then directly into the bowl of crumbs. Transfer your chops to a baking sheet. Lightly spray a little more oil on top of the pork and bake in the oven for 30 minutes.

Serves: 6   **Prep Time: 20 mins.**   **Cook Time: 30 mins.**
Calories: 378   **Protein: 33g**   **Carbs: 8g**   **Fat: 13g**

85. Crock Pot Asian Pork with Mushrooms

Ingredients

pork sirloin roast, 2 lb., lean, boneless
kosher salt and fresh cracked pepper
non-stick oil spray
chicken broth, 1 cup, fat-free, low-sodium
soy sauce, ½ cup, low sodium
balsamic vinegar, 1/ 3 cup
Stevia, 3 tbsp.
Cayenne and sesame oil, 1 tsp.

Chinese five spice, ½ tsp.
Garlic, 3 cloves, crushed
ginger root, 1 tbsp., grated
mushrooms, 8 oz., sliced
For Topping:
Scallions, ¼ cup, chopped
Cilantro, ¼ cup, chopped

Directions

Season the pork. Heat a skillet on medium-high heat spray with a little oil and brown pork for about 7-8 minutes. Add your ginger, garlic, five spice, sesame oil, agave, vinegar, soy sauce and broth into your slow cooker. Toss in the pork then set to low and cook for 8 hours. Take the pork out with 30 minutes before the time ends and allow the pork to rest. Toss in your mushrooms, cover and cook for about 30 minutes. Shred the pork and set to the side to re add once your mushrooms are cooked. Once the mushrooms have been cooked remove a cup of the broth and add in your pork and mix. Add your spinach at the very end, cover until it wilts. Serve.

Serves: 7   **Prep Time: 20 mins.**   **Cook Time: 8 hrs.**
Calories: 224.1   **Protein: 25g**   **Carbs: 11g**   **Fat: 8.5g**

86. Shrimp Scampi

Ingredients

1 package of angel hair pasta
½ cup of butter, melted
4 cloves of minced garlic
1 pound of shrimp

1 cup of dry white wine
¼ teaspoon of ground black pepper
¾ of grated Parmesan cheese
1 tablespoon of fresh parsley

Directions

Bring a pot of salted water to boil then add the pasta cook until just tender. Drain well. Add your butter into a saucepan on medium heat then add in your shrimp and garlic. Cook while stirring for about 4 minutes. Add in pepper and wine then stir. Allow to boil for about 30 seconds. Stir constantly then mix with drained pasta sprinkle with cheese and parsley on top.

Serves: 6   **Prep Time: 15 mins.**   **Cook Time: 5 mins.**
Calories: 268   **Protein: 19.7g**   **Carbs: 1.2g**   **Fat: 20.3g**

87. Dijon Salmon

Ingredients

4 fillets of salmon

3 tablespoons of Dijon mustard salt and pepper to taste

¼ cup of Italian styled bread crumbs

¼ cup of melted butter

Directions

Preheat oven to 400 and line a baking pan with aluminum foil. Place the skin side down of the salmon fillets spread a thin layer of mustard on top of each fillet, season with bread crumbs and drizzle with melted butter. Set to bake for about 15 minutes, your salmon should be flaky.

Serves: 4	**Prep Time: 8 mins.**	**Cook Time: 15 mins.**
Calories: 109	**Protein: 0.4g**	**Carbs: 1.4g** **Fat: 11.6g**

88. Broiled Tilapia Parmesan

Ingredients

Parmesan cheese, ½ cup

butter, ¼ cup, softened

mayonnaise, 3 tbsp.

lemon juice, 2 tbsp.

basil, ¼ tsp.

black pepper, ¼ tsp.

celery salt, 1/8 tsp.

Tilapia fillets, 2 lbs.

onion powder, ¼ tsp.

Directions

Set your broiler to preheat and line a broiling pan with aluminum foil. Combine your lemon juice, mayonnaise, butter and parmesan cheese in a bowl. Toss in your celery salt, onion powder, pepper, and dried basil then set aside. Arrange fillets in a single layer in pan broil for 3 minutes flip fillets and broil for another few minutes. Remove from oven cover with Parmesan cheese mixture then broil for another 2 minutes until top is browned.

Serves: 4	**Prep Time: 15 mins.**	**Cook Time: 5 mins.**
Calories: 414	**Protein: 50.1g**	**Carbs: 3.4g** **Fat: 22.5g**

89. Tuna Casserole

Ingredients

1 package of egg noodles

2 cups of frozen green peas

2 cans of mushroom soup

2 cans of tuna drained

1 onion chopped

10 slices of processed cheese black pepper to taste

Directions

Set a decent sized pot on with water and allow to boil. Once boiling, add in peas and noodles. Allow to cook until the noodles are fork tender, then drain. Return your peas and noodles to the pot. Mix pepper, cheese, onions, tuna and soup. Cook, while stirring, until your cheese melts.

Serves: 4	**Prep Time: 10 mins.**	**Cook Time: 7 mins.**
Calories: 139	**Protein: 20.1g**	**Carbs: 13.1g** **Fat: 1.1g**

90. Lemon Shrimp Linguine

Ingredients

1 package of linguine pasta
1 tablespoon of olive oil
6 cloves of garlic minced
½ cup of chicken broth
¼ cup of white wine
1 lemon juiced

½ teaspoon of lemon zest salt to taste
2 teaspoons of freshly ground black pepper
1 pound of fresh shrimp peeled and deveined
¼ cup butter
3 tablespoons of fresh chopped parsley
1 tablespoon chopped fresh basil

Directions

Set your slightly salted water to boil. Add in your noodles and allow to cook for 9 minutes then drain. Add your oil on medium heat and allow to get hot then sauté your garlic for a minute. Add in your pepper, salt, lemon zest, lemon juice, wine and chicken broth. Switch the heat to low and allow to simmer until liquid is reduced by ½. Mix basil, parsley, butter and shrimp into the saucepan. Cook for about 3 minutes so that your shrimp becomes opaque. Add back your linguine and allow to continue cooking until well cooked.

Serves: 4   **Prep Time: 10 mins.**   **Cook Time: 7 mins.**
Calories: 304   **Protein: 30.3g**   **Carbs: 2.9g**   **Fat: 18.6g**

PREDIABETES DINNER RECIPES

91. Edamame Veggie Burgers

Ingredients:

1 tablespoon plus 1 teaspoon canola oil
2 cups shiitake mushrooms, sliced
1 cup frozen shelled edamame, unthawed
1 clove garlic, roughly chopped
¾ cup shelled & peeled walnuts
1 tablespoon fresh parsley, roughly chopped

1 egg
1 teaspoon low sodium tamari or soy sauce
⅛ teaspoon ground ginger
⅛ teaspoon cumin
¼ cup whole wheat panko bread crumbs
½ teaspoon freshly ground black pepper

Directions:

Heat 1 teaspoon of oil in a small fry pan over medium-high heat, add mushrooms. Sauté until mushrooms are just softened, 3 to 5 minutes. In a food processor, combine mushrooms, edamame, garlic, walnuts, parsley, egg, tamari, ginger, cumin, panko and pepper. Process 30 minutes or until edamame and walnuts are finely chopped (don't over process or you may get a paste). Heat remaining oil in a large skillet heat over medium heat. Add burgers. Cook until golden brown on each side, turning once, about 5 to 7 minutes. Serve immediately.

Serves: 4	Prep Time: 15 mins.		Cooking Time: 42 mins.
Calories: 300	Protein: 12g	Carbs: 21g	Fat: 20g

92. Vegetarian Reuben Sandwich

Ingredients:

2 teaspoons extra virgin olive oil, plus 1 teaspoon
½ cup chopped onion
1 sliced portabella mushroom
4 ounces seitan, drained and thinly sliced
½ teaspoon garlic powder
⅛ teaspoon kosher salt
⅛ teaspoon freshly ground pepper

1 tablespoon mayonnaise (olive-oil based one)
1 teaspoon ketchup
1 teaspoon finely chopped dill pickle
2 slices sprouted grain bread
2 tablespoons sauerkraut, drained
1-ounce Swiss cheese

Directions:

In a large skillet, add 2 teaspoons of olive oil and onions. Cook over medium heat until almost caramelized, about 10 minutes. Add portabella mushroom slices, seitan, garlic powder, salt, and pepper. Mix well. Cook for 4 to 6 minutes, until seitan and mushrooms are cooked and onions are caramelized. To make dressing, whisk together mayonnaise, ketchup, and pickle in small bowl.

Heat grill pan over medium-high heat. Lightly brush each slice of bread with remaining olive oil on one side. Pile the seitan, onions and mushrooms on the bread (greased side down). Drizzle sandwich with dressing. Top with sauerkraut followed by cheese. Top with another slice of bread (greased side up). Place on grill. Cook until cheese is melted and bread is toasted, about 2 to 3 minutes on each side.

Serves: 1	Prep Time: 15 mins.		Cooking Time: 22 mins.
Calories: 448	Protein: 23g	Carbs: 26g	Fat: 29g

93. Ultimate Vegetable Sandwich

Ingredients

2 tablespoons extra virgin olive oil, divided
Zucchini, 1 small, sliced in an angle
4 lengthwise strips of red pepper
1 small yellow squash, sliced in an angle
4 slices red onion
¼ teaspoon kosher salt
½ teaspoon freshly ground black pepper

4 slices sourdough bread
½ cup arugula
6 ounces fresh water-packed
mozzarella cheese,
drained, sliced
1 tablespoon Walnut Pesto

Directions

Heat a grill pan over medium-high heat. Using a pastry brush, brush half of oil on both sides of the zucchini, squash, red pepper, and onion slices. Season with salt and pepper. Transfer your vegetables to a hot grill then allow to cook until they are tender. Cool completely. Once vegetables are done, brush bread slices with olive oil and grill on both sides.

Spread pesto on one side of bread slices. To assemble sandwiches, start with the bottom 2 slices of bread (pesto side up). On each, place arugula, stack 2 slices of zucchini, 2 slices of squash, 2 slices of red pepper, and onion. Top with mozzarella. Add the remaining bread slices on top with the pesto side facing down.

Serves: 4	**Prep Time: 15 mins.**		**Cooking Time: 8 mins.**
Calories: 625	**Protein: 36g**	**Carbs: 45g**	**Fat: 36g**

94. Steak Tacos

Ingredients

8 large lettuce leaves
3 Tablespoons olive oil
1 pound skirt steak or flank steak
½ bunch cilantro, chopped

8 radishes, chopped
4 scallions, chopped
1 teaspoon sea salt

Directions

Set your oil oh high heat to get hot. Set the steak to cook for about 10 minutes, flipping half way. Wash the lettuce and pat the leaves dry with paper towels. In a bowl, combine the radishes, scallions, cilantro, lime juice, and 2 Tablespoons of olive oil. Fill each of the lettuce leaves with the steak and top with the radish mixture.

Serves: 4	**Prep Time: 10 mins.**		**Cooking Time: 10 mins.**
Calories: 677	**Protein: 47.6g**	**Carbs: 73.7g**	**Fat: 26.6g**

95. Skillet Sausage Scramble

Ingredients

2 Tablespoons coconut oil

1 small yellow onion, diced

16 ounces sausage, chopped

1 large sweet potato, peeled and diced

2 cups baby spinach

¼ cup water

Sea salt to taste

½ teaspoon cinnamon (optional)

Directions

Sauté the onion in the oil in a large skillet over medium-high heat until just starting to brown, about 5 minutes. Add the sausage and sauté until browned, about 10 minutes. Add the sweet potato, water, and cinnamon (if using). Cover and cook until the sweet potato is tender, 10-15 minutes. Remove cover and stir in spinach. Stir until spinach is wilted.

Serves: 4	Prep Time: 10 mins.		Cooking Time: 35 mins.
Calories: 402	Protein: 22.6 g	Carbs: 22.9g	Fat: 27.5g

96. Quick Chicken Stir-Fry

Ingredients

1-pound chicken meat, cut into 1-inch chunks

1 yellow onion, sliced

2 carrots, peeled and sliced thinly

4 cups baby bok choy (about 2 heads), chopped

12 ounces mushrooms, halved

4 Tablespoons coconut oil

4 cloves garlic, chopped

1 Tablespoon grated ginger

1 Tablespoon apple cider vinegar.

1 teaspoon sea salt

Directions

Sauté onions in coconut oil in a deep sauté pan or wok for about 3 minutes, or until translucent. Add in your chicken and allow to cook, while stirring, until lightly browned. Add the bok choy, carrots, and mushrooms and continue to sauté for a few minutes. In a separate bowl, mix the vinegar, garlic, ginger, and salt, and whisk until blended. Pour the sauce over the chicken and vegetables and cook, stirring frequently until vegetables are crisp-tender.

Serves: 4	Prep Time: 15 mins.		Cooking Time: 20 mins.
Calories: 321	Protein: 25.2 g	Carbs: 4.2g	Fat: 23.1g

97. Turkey Lasagna

Ingredients

1-pound ground turkey
4 large zucchini, sliced thinly lengthwise
1 yellow onion, chopped
2 cups mushrooms, sliced
2 cups baby spinach

2 cups fresh basil
1 lemon, juiced (about 2 Tablespoons)
¼ cup olive oil, plus 2 Tablespoon
1 clove garlic
1 teaspoon sea salt

Directions

Preheat the oven to 425 °F. Sauté onions in 1 Tablespoon olive oil in a deep sauté pan or wok for about 3 minutes, or until translucent. Add the mushrooms and turkey and cook, stirring frequently, until lightly browned. While chicken is cooking, combine spinach, basil, coconut, lemon juice, ¼ cup olive oil, garlic, and salt in a food processor and process 30-45 seconds, until combined but still coarse. Grease the bottom of an 8 x 10 inch baking pan with 1 Tablespoon of the oil. Layer one-third of the zucchini slices on the bottom. Top with one-third of the turkey mixture, then one-third of the sauce. Repeat the layers twice more, ending with the sauce on top. Bake about 30 minutes.

Serves: 4	**Prep Time: 20 mins.**		**Cooking Time: 20 mins.**
Calories: 709	**Protein: 23.2 g**	**Carbs: 4.2g**	**Fat: 66.5g**

98. Coconut-Crusted Cod

Ingredients

1-pound fresh cod fillets, cut into 4 pieces
½ cup unsweetened coconut milk
½ cup unsweetened shredded coconut

½ teaspoon ground ginger
1 teaspoon sea salt
1 Tablespoon coconut oil

Directions

Preheat oven to 400 °F. Place the coconut milk in one shallow bowl and the shredded coconut, salt, and ginger in another. Dip the fish in the milk, then dredge each side in the coconut, and place it on a baking sheet, greased with coconut oil. Bake 15 minutes, until fish is flaky and cooked through.

Serves: 2	**Prep Time: 10 mins.**		**Cooking Time: 15 mins.**
Calories: 867	**Protein: 54 g**	**Carbs: 26.3g**	**Fat: 62.1g**

99. Delicious Lobster Bisque

Ingredients

16 oz (1 lb.) lobster meat (claws and tail from 2 - 3 lobsters)
4 cups vegetable broth
1 can (13.5 oz) full-fat coconut milk (or lite coconut milk)
1 can (6 oz) organic tomato paste
2 tbsp. coconut aminos (apple cider vinegar or liquid aminos)
2 leeks
2 carrots
2 celery stalks

4 large garlic cloves
2 bay leaves
1/2 tsp. dried basil
1/2 tsp. dried thyme
1 tsp. dried oregano
1 tsp. black pepper
Celtic sea salt, to taste
1 small bunch parsley (for garnish)
2 tbsp. ghee (or bacon fat, cacao butter, or coconut oil)

Directions

Chop leeks, carrots and celery. Peel garlic and chop. Add to medium pot with vegetable broth, oregano, basil, thyme, pepper and salt to taste. Add tomato paste and stir to combine. Simmer about 25 minutes. Bring large pot salted water to boil. Boil each lobster about 2 minutes. Let cool, then crack shells and remove meat from claws and tail. Roughly chop and set aside. Pour veggies and broth into food processor or high-speed blender. Process until puréed, about 2 minutes. Add puréed mixture back to pot and heat over medium heat. Bring to simmer and add chopped lobster meat. Stir to combine. Simmer until lobster is cooked through and tender, about 10 minutes. Transfer to serving dish and serve hot.

Serves: 4	Prep Time: 25 mins.		Cooking Time: 40 mins.
Calories: 867	Protein: 54 g	Carbs: 26.3g	Fat: 62.1g

100. Ethiopian Beef Stew

Ingredients

stew beef, 24 oz
beef stock, 2 cups
2 tablespoons organic tomato paste
raw honey, 1/2 tsp.
onion, 1 small
garlic, 2 cloves
Celtic sea salt, 2 tsp.
Spice Blend, 2 tsp.
Ghee, 2 tbsp.
coconut oil, 3 tbsp.

Spice Blend

Nutmeg, 1/8 tsp., ground
Allspice, 1/8 tsp., ground

Turmeric, 1/8 tsp.
Cumin, 1/4 tsp., ground
Cinnamon, 1/4 tsp., ground
Cloves, 1/4 tsp., ground
garlic powder, 1/4 tsp.
black pepper, 1/2 tsp., ground
fenugreek, 1/2 tsp., ground
ginger, 1/2 tsp., ground
coriander, 1/2 tsp., ground
cardamom seed, 1/2 tsp.
onion flakes, 1 tsp. dried
paprika, 1 tbsp.
red pepper flakes, 2 tbsp.

Directions

Heat medium pot over medium-high heat. Add Spice blend and toast until fragrant. Stir frequently and do not burn. Remove toasted Spice Blend and set aside. Add ghee and coconut oil to hot pot. Cut beef into 1-inch chunks. Set aside. Peel onion and garlic. Mince garlic and dice onion.

Add to hot oiled pot and sauté until caramelized, about 2 - 3 minutes. Add tomato paste, 2 teaspoons Spice Blend and honey to pot. Stir and cook into thick paste, about 2 minutes. Stir in a few tablespoons of beef stock to loosen paste.

Add beef, remaining beef stock and salt to pot. Stir to combine. Reduce heat to medium-low and simmer until beef is tender and sauce thickens and reduces, about 1 hour. Stir occasionally. Transfer to serving dish and serve room temperature.

Serves: 4	Prep Time: 30 mins.		Cooking Time: 1 hr.
Calories: 383	Protein: 38.6 g	Carbs: 7.7g	Fat: 23.2g

101. Stewed Chicken and Dumplings

Ingredients

Chicken, 2 lb., whole, innards removed
Water, 6 - 10 cups
Carrots, 3
celery, 3 stalks
white onion, 1 small
bay leaves, 4
Thyme, 1 ½ tsp., dried
Oregano, ½ tsp., dried
Paprika, 1 tsp.
black pepper, 2 tsp.
Celtic sea salt, 1 tbsp.

almond flour, 3 cups
arrowroot powder, ½ cup
Eggs, 2, cage-free
coconut oil, ½ cup, chilled
baking soda, ½ tsp.
Bay leaf, ¼ tsp., ground
Thyme, 1 tsp., dried
white pepper, 1/2 tsp., ground
Celtic sea salt, 1 tsp.
Nut milk

Dumplings

Directions

Heat large pot over medium-high heat. Place chicken breast-down in hot pot. Sear chicken and turn to brown and render out fat for about 15 minutes. Chop carrots and celery. Peel onion and mince. Add to chicken with salt and spices. Sauté about 2 minutes.

Add enough water to pot to cover chicken. Switch the heat up to high and allow to boil. Once boiling, switch the heat to medium then allow to simmer for about 30 minutes. Place lid loosely over pot to prevent splatter, if necessary. For Dumplings, sift almond flour and arrowroot into medium mixing bowl. Cut in solid oil or butter with fork until crumbly mixture forms.

Add egg, salt and spices, baking soda, and enough nut milk or chicken broth from pot to bring together soft, slightly sticky dough. Carefully remove chicken from pot with long utensil and set aside. Use utensils to remove skin from chicken. Carve chicken into desired pieces and place back in back. Use spoon or scoop to gently drop dough into pot.

Cover with well-fitting lid and let simmer about 15 - 20 minutes, until Dumplings and chicken are cooked through. Gently stir soup to periodically prevent Dumplings from sticking. Turn over any Dumplings that are not submerged. Remove from heat and transfer to serving dish. Serve hot.

Serves: 4	Prep Time: 10 mins.		Cooking Time: 1 hr. 20 mins.
Calories: 537	Protein: 47.9 g	Carbs: 10.4g	Fat: 34.2g

102. Indian Egg Fried Rice

Ingredients

1/2 head cauliflower, minced
4 cage-free eggs
2 tablespoons pure fish sauce
1 small carrot
1/2 red bell pepper
1/2 yellow bell pepper
1/4 onion
2 small green onions

1 tablespoon coconut Aminos
1 teaspoon sesame oil (optional)
1 large garlic clove
1/2 piece fresh ginger
1/2 teaspoon red pepper flake
Celtic sea salt, to taste
Bacon fat or coconut oil (for cooking)
Water

Directions

Heat medium pan or wok over high heat. Lightly coat with bacon fat or coconut oil. Whisk eggs in medium mixing bowl. Set aside.

Remove stems, seeds and veins from bell peppers, then julienne (thinly slice). Finely dice carrot. Slice green onions. Peel and mince garlic, ginger and onion. Add red pepper flakes to hot oiled pan. Sauté until just cooked fragrant, about 30 seconds. Add garlic, ginger and onion and sauté about 1 minute.

Add cauliflower to hot pan. Sauté about 5 minutes, until cauliflower is golden and a bit softened. Add carrot, peppers and 1/2 green onions. Cook another 2 - 5 minutes, until cauliflower is cooked through. Add a few tablespoons of water and cover with lid to steam, if desired. Arrange the vegetables to form a well in the center of the pan.

Pour whisked eggs into well in center and carefully scramble until fully cooked, about 2 minutes. Mix eggs into veggies. Remove from heat and transfer to serving dish. Top with green onions and serve.

Serves: 2	Prep Time: 10 mins.	Cooking Time: 15 mins.
Calories: 115	Protein: 4.4 g Carbs: 20.8g	Fat: 2.8g

103. Sliced Veggie Spicy Chicken

Ingredients

4 pieces grass-fed chicken thighs
1 onion
2 cloves garlic
3/4 cup sliced carrots
2 handfuls Kale greens
2 tbsp Chinese five spice

2 tbsp smoked paprika
2 tbsp chipotle chili pepper powder
1 tbsp olive oil
2 tsp lemon juice
1 tbsp coconut oil
4 cups water

Directions

Mince garlic and chop onion to desired size (medium strips work best). Chop carrots to 1/4" thickness. De-rib the kale and chop it coarsely, wash it and allow water to remain on the leaves. Add water to a pot and allow to lightly boil. Set your oil on medium heat to get hot. Add carrot and onion and cook for 8 minutes, stirring occasionally. Meanwhile, heat 1 tbsp coconut oil over medium heat in a separate pan. Add chicken and cook for 4 minutes.

Season chicken with Chinese five spice, chipotle chili pepper powder and smoked paprika and turn, adding more of each spice to the other side of the chicken, cooking for another 4 minutes or until cooked through. Add kale to boiling water and boil until bright green, about 5 minutes. Remove from water and let sit while the vegetables and chicken continue cooking. Add everything into the pan with the vegetables and add 2 tsp lemon juice. Add minced garlic and stir for 1 minute. Serve immediately.

Serves: 4	Prep Time: 4 mins.		Cooking Time: 8 mins.
Calories: 87	Protein: 1.1 g	Carbs: 5.9g	Fat: 7.3g

104. Spicy Kale Quiche

Ingredients

Eggs, 8, cage-free
Olive oil, 2 tbsp., extra virgin
Kale greens, 7 oz., washed, trimmed
Shallot, 1, minced
chipotle chili pepper powder, ¼ tsp.

garlic, 2 cloves, minced
lemon, ½, juiced
coconut oil, 2 tbsp.
black pepper, ¼ tbsp., ground

Directions

Fit your steamer basket into a pot then fill it with water. Allow the water to boil. Add your kale into the water and allow to steam until forest green. Set a large pot on then add your eggs and oil. Add in chili pepper and scramble. Transfer your kale to the eggs then add in your lemon juice, shallots and garlic. Top with coconut oil evenly then season with black pepper. Stir well and serve.

Serves: 4	Prep Time: 10 mins.		Cooking Time: 15 mins.
Calories: 91	Protein: 0.3 g	Carbs: 1.2g	Fat: 9.8g

105. No-Bun Nuts & Turkey Burgers

Ingredients

16 oz ground turkey
1 cup walnuts
2 cloves garlic
1 onion
¼ tsp chipotle chili pepper powder

¼ tbsp smoked paprika
¼ tsp ground black pepper
Lettuce leaves
Sliced tomatoes

Directions

Chop walnuts into smaller pieces, about ⅛" cubes. Mince garlic and chop onion into small pieces, about ¼" pieces. Combine the above with ground turkey and add chipotle chili pepper powder, smoked paprika and ground black pepper. Knead it all together and separate into four patties. Cook on the grill on high heat, flipping occasionally, until desired done-ness. Serve with lettuce leaves and tomato slices.

Serves: 4	**Prep Time: 10 mins.**		**Cooking Time: 6-12 mins.**
Calories: 694	**Protein: 25.18 g**	**Carbs: 6.5g**	**Fat: 63.6g**

106. Chicken Bruschetta

Ingredients

4 grass-fed chicken breasts
2 tomatoes
4 olives
2 onions

¼ tsp ground black pepper
1 cup roasted red pepper
3 tbsp extra virgin olive oil

Directions

Dice the tomatoes, chop the olives and onions, and combine them with ground black pepper and 2 tbsp olive oil in a bowl and mix well into a bruschetta. Puree the roasted red pepper in a blender and set aside. Combine the chicken with 1 tbsp extra virgin olive oil and cook in a pan over medium-high heat for 4 minutes, turn once, and cook another 4-6 minutes, removing from heat while still tender. Place one piece of chicken on each plate and pour the roasted red pepper over each, adding bruschetta over the top. Garnish with basil and serve.

Serves: 4	**Prep Time: 10 mins.**		**Cooking Time: 10 mins.**
Calories: 88	**Protein: 1.6g**	**Carbs: 10.2g**	**Fat: 5.2g**

107. Chick-Plant Filets

Ingredients

4 grass-fed chicken breasts
1 eggplant
4 pinches fresh basil
¼ tsp chipotle chili pepper powder
¼ tsp curry

1 large carrot
1 red onion
1 cup coconut milk
8 wooden toothpicks
1 tbsp coconut oil

Directions

Cut eggplant into 8 rectangles 3" long by 1" wide and 1" tall. Cut the carrot into matchsticks and dice the onion into small pieces. Cut the chicken in half lengthwise into thin filets. Soak the toothpicks in water. Preheat oven to 350. Combine coconut oil, carrot, onion, 1 tsp curry, basil and chipotle chili pepper powder in a pan over medium heat. Stir together until it forms a sauce. Add eggplant and sauté 7-10 minutes or until eggplant is tender. Place 1 slice of eggplant on each of the chicken filets. Drizzle the contents of the pan over each of the filets; roll each fillet up around the eggplant and secure with a toothpick. Place the 8 filets in the oven and bake for 35 minutes. Remove from oven and pour serve 2 filets to each plate. Pour ¼ cup coconut milk and sprinkle curry over each plate's filets. Chill 20 minutes and then serve.

Serves: 4	Prep Time: 10 mins.		Cooking Time: 50 mins.
Calories: 120	Protein: 3.8g	Carbs: 15.4g	Fat: 5.7g

108. All-Day Meatball Marinara

Ingredients

24 oz (1 1/2 lbs) ground meat (ground beef, pork, turkey, or any combination)
1/2 cup almond meal (or finely ground almonds)
2 cage-free eggs
2 cans (15 oz) organic tomato sauce
1 can (15 oz) organic crushed tomatoes
1/4 cup nutritional yeast (optional)
1 small onion (yellow or white)
2 garlic cloves
1 bay leaf

2 sprigs fresh basil
3 teaspoons dried oregano
2 teaspoons dried parsley
1 teaspoon dried basil
1/2 teaspoon onion powder
1/2 teaspoon garlic powder
1 teaspoon Celtic sea salt
1 tablespoon coconut oil (for cooking)
1 small bunch fresh flat-leaf Italian parsley (for garnish)

Directions

Heat large skillet over medium-high heat. Add coconut oil to hot pan. Peel onion and cut in half. Finely grate one half and add to medium mixing bowl. Reserve second half. Peel and mince garlic. Add half to mixing bowl. Reserve second half.

Add ground meat to medium mixing bowl with 1/4 cup tomato sauce, almond meal, eggs, 1 teaspoon dried oregano, 1 teaspoon dried parsley, onion powder, garlic powder, 1/2 teaspoon salt, and nutritional yeast (optional). Mix until well combined. Form mixture into medium-sized meat balls. Add to hot oiled pan in batches and brown on all sides, about 5 minute per batch. Set aside in slow cooker.

Finely chop remaining onions. Add to hot oiled pan with garlic. Sauté about 5 minutes. Add remaining tomato sauce, crushed tomatoes, 2 teaspoons dried oregano, 1 teaspoon dried parsley, 1/2 teaspoon salt, bay leaf, and fresh torn basil leaves.

Stir and bring to simmer, about 5 minutes. Pour sauce over meatballs and stir to combine. Cover slow cooker with lid. Turn on to low and cook 4 - 5 hours, until meatballs are cooked through. Turn off slow cooker and carefully remove lid. Transfer to serving dish. For garnish, chop fresh parsley and sprinkle over dish. Serve hot.

Serves: 4   Prep Time: 20 mins.   Cooking Time: 4 hrs.
Calories: 927   Protein: 36.5g   Carbs: 61.6g   Fat: 55.8g

109. Natural Italian Chicken Sausage

Ingredients

20 oz (1 1/4 lb.) chicken (ground meat or whole pieces)
1/2 teaspoon all spice
1 teaspoon fennel seed
1 teaspoon ground sage
1 teaspoon dried thyme

1 teaspoon ground black pepper
1 teaspoon Celtic sea salt
Natural or synthetic sausage casing (optional)
Piping or kitchen bag (optional)
Coconut oil (for cooking)

Directions

Heat medium skillet over medium heat and lightly coat with coconut oil. Remove chicken skin and bones from pieces and coarsely grind in food processor, high-speed blender or meat grinder, if using. Add ground chicken to medium mixing bowl with salt and spices and mix well. Use meat grinder to stuff mixture into casing. Or scoop mixture into piping bag with no tip or kitchen bag with 1 inch corner cut off, and pipe into casing. Twist casing tightly in opposite directions to section off 4-inch links while stuffing. Or form into 8 - 12 round patties with hands. Place links or patties in hot oiled skillet. Cook links about 4 - 5 minutes per side, until golden brown and cooked through. Or cook patties about 3 - 4 minutes per side, until golden brown and crisp. Turn halfway through cooking. Drain cooked sausage on paper towel. Serve hot.

Serves: 4	Prep Time: 5 mins.		Cooking Time: 10 mins.
Calories: 927	Protein: 36.5g	Carbs: 61.6g	Fat: 55.8g

110. Ground Beef Stuffed Peppers

Ingredients

4 bell peppers
16 oz (1 lb) ground meat (beef, pork, chicken, turkey, etc.)
1/2 head cauliflower (1 cup riced)
1/2 cup roasted red peppers
1/4 cup sundried tomatoes
1/4 cup pecans
1/2 small onion (white, yellow or red)

2 tablespoons coconut oil
2 garlic cloves
Medium bunch fresh herbs (parsley, oregano, thyme, etc.)
1/4 teaspoon red pepper flakes
1 teaspoon ground white pepper (or black pepper)
1 teaspoon Celtic sea salt
Water

Directions

Preheat oven to 350 degrees F. Cut tops off peppers, then remove stems from tops and seeds and veins from bottoms of peppers. Leave bottoms of peppers hollow but do not pierce. Place in baking dish just large enough to fit peppers snuggly. Set aside. Peel onion and garlic. Roughly chop onions, garlic and cauliflower. Add to food processor or high-speed blender with pecans. Pulse about 15 seconds. Add tops of peppers, roasted red peppers, sundried tomatoes, ground meat, salt, pepper, and fresh herbs to processor. Process until coarsely ground, about 1 - 2 minutes. Use large spoon to stuff peppers with mixture. Add about a half cup of water to your baking dish. Cover peppers with aluminum foil. Bake 30 minutes. Carefully remove foil and continue baking uncovered 10 - 20 minutes, until stuffing is golden brown and cooked through. Carefully remove from oven and transfer peppers to serving dish. Serve hot.

Serves: 4	Prep Time: 10 mins.		Cooking Time: 50 mins.
Calories: 518	Protein: 18.9g	Carbs: 10g	Fat: 45.6g

111. Healthy Gyro with Creamy Tzatziki

Ingredients

2 large romaine lettuce leaves
1 tomato
1/2 small red onion

Gyro Meat

8 oz (1/2 lb) ground lamb
8 oz (1/2 lb) ground beef
1 small onion (white or yellow)
2 garlic cloves
1 teaspoon dried marjoram
1 teaspoon dried oregano
1 teaspoon dried rosemary
1 teaspoon ground black pepper

1 teaspoon Celtic sea salt
Coconut oil (for cooking)

Coconut Cream Tzatziki

1/2 small cucumber
1/4 cup coconut cream (settled from full-fat canned coconut milk)
1 teaspoon lemon juice
1/2 teaspoon apple cider vinegar
2 mint leaves
1 sprig fresh dill
1 garlic clove
1/4 teaspoon Celtic sea salt

Directions

Preheat oven to 325 degrees F. Line small loaf pan with parchment or aluminum foil. For Gyro Meat, peel white or yellow onion and add to food processor or high-speed blender. Process until finely ground, about 30 seconds. Turn out onto cheesecloth or paper towels. Squeeze or compress onions to remove as much liquid as possible. Add drained onions back to processor.

Peel garlic and add to processor with lamb, beef, herbs, salt and pepper. Process to make the mixture smooth, about 2 - 3 minutes. Scrape down sides of bowl as necessary. Add mixture to prepared loaf pan. Pack tightly and smooth top. Bake for 30 minutes. Switch the oven off and transfer your loaf pan to a cool place to rest for about 5 minutes. For Coconut Cream Tzatziki, peel, seed and shred, grate or dice cucumber. Peel and mince garlic.

Mince mint and dill. Add to small mixing bowl with coconut cream, lemon juice, salt and vinegar. Mix well, then set aside to chill in refrigerator. Heat medium skillet over medium-high heat and lightly coat with coconut oil. Carefully release Gyro Meat from loaf pan and peel away parchment or aluminum. Use tongs and sharp knife to cut lengthwise into 1/4-inch-thick slices.

Add sliced meat to hot oiled skillet in single layer and sear about 2 minutes on each side, until browned and lightly crisp. Flip halfway through cooking. Peel and slice red onion. Seed and chop tomato. Transfer romaine lettuce to serving dishes. Layer Gyro Meat over lettuce, then top with Coconut Cream Tzatziki, onions and tomatoes. Use lettuce to wrap up meat and veggies and serve immediately.

Serves: 2   **Prep Time: 10 mins.**   **Cooking Time: 30 mins.**
Calories: 870   **Protein: 49.9g**   **Carbs: 39.6g**   **Fat: 60g**

112. Chicken Souvlaki Kebobs

Ingredients

12 oz (3/4 lb.) boneless skinless chicken
1 lemon
2 garlic cloves
1/2 small white onion
1/2 yellow bell pepper

1/2 cup grape tomato
1 teaspoon dried oregano
3/4 teaspoon Celtic sea salt
2 tablespoons coconut oil
8 skewers

Directions

Soak wooden skewers in water for 10 minutes, if using. Juice lemon into medium mixing bowl. Peel and mince garlic. Remove stem, seeds and veins from bell pepper. Peel onion. Roughly chop pepper and onion. Add to bowl with tomatoes, 1 tablespoon coconut oil, oregano and salt. Pierce chicken multiple times with fork, then cut into one inch chunks.

Add to bowl and mix to combine. Let set aside in refrigerator for 10 minutes. Heat small skillet or griddle over medium-high heat and add 1 tablespoon coconut oil. Drain marinated chicken and veggies, then carefully add to skewer, alternating meat and veggies. Add chicken and veggie skewer to hot oiled skillet or griddle. Grill for about 1 - 2 minutes then turn 1/4 the way around. Continue cooking and turning until chicken is golden brown and cooked through. Remove from heat and serve immediately.

Serves: 4	Prep Time: 5 mins.		Cooking Time: 15 mins.
Calories: 189	Protein: 19.76g	Carbs: 7.2g	Fat: 9.2g

113. Macadamia Crusted Ahi Tuna

Ingredients

8 oz ahi tuna fillet
1/4 teaspoon coconut oil
1/4 teaspoon dried thyme
1/4 teaspoon dried tarragon (optional)
1/4 cup whole macadamia nuts (shelled)
1 small garlic clove teaspoon

1 small shallot teaspoon
1/2 teaspoon ground white pepper (or black pepper)
1/2 teaspoon sea salt
2 tablespoons coconut oil

Directions

Heat medium pan over medium-high heat. Add 2 tablespoons coconut oil to pan. Chop macadamia nuts well. Peel and finely mince garlic and shallot. Set aside. Rub top and bottom of fillet with 1/4 teaspoon coconut oil, salt, pepper, thyme and tarragon (optional). Press 1/2 chopped macadamia nuts into each side of fillet. Add garlic and shallots to hot oiled pan and sauté for just a second. Do not burn. Carefully place fish in pan and sear 15 - 30 seconds on each side, for rare to medium rare. Carefully flip half way through cooking. Transfer fillet to serving dish and serve hot with mixed greens or favorite veggies.

Serves: 2	Prep Time: 10 mins.		Cooking Time: 1 mins.
Calories: 371	Protein: 29.2g	Carbs: 3.4g	Fat: 27.4g

114. Insulin-Friendly Seafood Paella

Ingredients

1 large head cauliflower
8 oz chorizo (or other smoked sausage)
8 oz large shrimp
12 live little neck clams
12 live mussels
4 bone-in chicken thighs
1 cup chicken stock (or seafood stock)

1 small white onion
2 tablespoons smoked paprika
1 teaspoon saffron
Pinch ground black pepper
Pinch sea salt
2 tablespoons coconut oil

Directions

Set your oil on medium heat to get hot. Peel and chop onion. Add to hot oiled pan and sauté until translucent, about 2 minutes. Add chicken thighs and brown about 5 minutes. Turn chicken over and cook another 5 minutes. Rinse and clean clams and mussels, and remove any beards with pliers. Peel and devein shrimp. Cut chorizo into 1 inch slices. Set aside. Roughly chop cauliflower and add to food processor with shredding attachment, process to "rice." Or mince cauliflower with knife.

Add riced or minced cauliflower to chicken and sauté 2 minutes. Add chorizo, clams, mussels and shrimp. Add paprika and saffron and sauté another 2 minutes. Add chicken or seafood stock and stir to combine. Increase heat to high and bring to simmer. Reduce heat to medium-high and cover. Let simmer about 5 - 7 minutes, until liquid evaporates, shrimp is opaque, and mussels and clams open. Discard any that do not open. Plate and serve hot.

Serves: 4   Prep Time: 10 mins.   Cooking Time: 25 mins.
Calories: 638   Protein: 56g   Carbs: 11.7g   Fat: 40.4g

115. Chicken Pot Pie

Ingredients

Filling

8 oz skin-on chicken
1 1/2 cup chicken broth
2 tablespoons tapioca flour
2 tablespoons coconut oil
2 carrots
1 celery stalk
1 green bell pepper
1 small onion
2 garlic cloves
2 teaspoons dried thyme (or 4 teaspoons fresh thyme)

1 tablespoon lemon juice
1/2 teaspoon black pepper
Pinch sea salt

Crust

1/3 cup almond flour
2 tablespoons coconut flour
3 tablespoons cold coconut oil (or cacao butter)
1 egg
3 - 4 teaspoons water
1/2 teaspoon dried thyme
1/4 teaspoon sea salt

Directions

Preheat oven to 400 degrees F. Heat medium pot over medium heat. Add two tablespoon coconut oil to hot pot. Add chicken pieces skin side down. Cook about 3 minutes, then turn with tongs and continue cooking another 3 minutes. Remove chicken and set aside. Whisk coconut flour into pot until smooth. Gradually whisk in chicken broth. Simmer about 5 minutes, whisking occasionally. Peel and mince garlic. Chop carrots, celery, onion and bell pepper. Add to pot with thyme, salt pepper and lemon juice. Chop par-cooked chicken meat. Add back to pot and simmer for 5 minutes. Remove from heat and set aside. For Crust, add cold coconut oil to flours, thyme and salt in small bowl.

Cut fat into flour with fork until crumbly. Mix in egg and enough water to bring together tender dough. Divide dough into 4 portions. Roll into balls and flatten into round disks large enough to fit over mini pie tins or ceramic ramekins with hand, then rolling pin. Pour Filling into vessels and cover with crusts. Pinch edges of dough over edges of vessels to seal in liquid. Brush top of each pie with coconut oil, coconut milk, or egg wash and sprinkle with salt. Use knife to cut a slit in the top of each pie. Bake pot pies for about 15 minutes, until crust is golden. Switch the oven off and transfer the pies to a cool place to cool down for about 10 minutes. Serve warm. Or let cool completely and serve room temperature.

Serves: 4	Prep Time: 15 mins.		Cooking Time: 30 mins.
Calories: 518	Protein: 32.6g	Carbs: 12.3g	Fat: 37.39g

116. Asian Empanada

Ingredients

Crust
1 cup almond flour
1 cup coconut flour
2 eggs
3 tablespoons sesame oil (or coconut oil)
1/2 teaspoon garlic powder
1/2 teaspoon onion powder
1/2 teaspoon ground ginger
1/4 teaspoon baking soda
1 teaspoon sea salt
1 tablespoon sesame oil (or coconut oil)
1 tablespoon sesame seeds

Filling
6 oz chicken or shrimp
1/2 head cabbage (1 cup shredded)
1 carrot
1/4 cup mushrooms
2 inch piece fresh ginger
2 garlic cloves
1 tablespoon pure fish sauce
1 teaspoon apple cider vinegar
1 shallot
1 scallion
1 teaspoon sesame oil

Directions

For Crust, sift almond and coconut flour into medium mixing bowl. Add baking soda, spices and salt. Whisk eggs in small mixing bowl, then add to flour and combine. Slowly add 3 tablespoons oil until malleable dough comes together. Roll in plastic wrap or wrap tightly in parchment and refrigerate for 15 minutes. Preheat oven to 400 degrees. Line sheet pan with parchment or baking mat.

Cover cutting board with parchment. Heat medium pan over medium heat. Shred cabbage, grate carrot, slice mushrooms. Peel and grate ginger. Slice scallion. Peel and mince shallot and garlic. Dice chicken or slice shrimp in half. Add sesame oil to pan. Add chicken or shrimp hot oiled pan with ginger, shallot and garlic. Sauté about 90 seconds. Add cabbage, carrot, and mushrooms and sauté for a minute.

Add vinegar and fish sauce. Sauté about 3 minutes until cabbage is wilted. Stir in scallions. Remove from heat and set aside. Remove dough from refrigerator. Divide dough into 4 portions. Roll dough into balls and flatten on parchment covered cutting board with hands. Roll into circles about 1/8-inch-thick with rolling pin. Scoop equal portions of Filling into center of one side of dough circle. Fold bare half of dough over filled half. Press edges together, letting any trapped air escape.

Crimp edges of dough together with fork. Repeat with remaining dough. Bruch tops of empanada with sesame oil and sprinkle with sesame seeds. Arrange empanadas on lined sheet pan and bake 15 - 20 minutes, or until dough is golden and cooked through. Serve immediately.

Serves: 4   **Prep Time: 20 mins.**   **Cooking Time: 20 mins.**
Calories: 319   **Protein: 14.7g**   **Carbs: 11.6g**   **Fat: 24.7g**

117. Zucchini Pasta with Pesto

Ingredients

1 small zucchini

1 bell pepper (or 1 carrot)

Pine Nut Pesto

2 1/2 cups fresh basil leaves

1/2 cup raw pine nuts

1 garlic clove

2 tbsp. raw oil

1/4 tsp. white pepper

1/4 tsp. Celtic sea salt

Directions

Carefully slice zucchini with spiralizer, vegetable peeler, or sharp knife. Carefully slice carrot with spiralizer, vegetable peeler, or grater, if using. Or remove stem, seeds and veins from bell pepper, then julienne (cut into long thin slices). Set aside. For Pine Nut Pesto, peel garlic and add to food processor or high-speed blender with basil, 2 tablespoons pine nuts, oil, salt and pepper. Process until thick, smooth mixture forms, about 1 - 2 minutes. Add Pine Nut Pesto to veggie pasta and toss to coat. Transfer to serving dish and top with remaining pine nuts. Serve immediately.

Serves: 2	**Prep Time: 10 mins.**	**Cooking Time: 0 mins.**
Calories: 361	**Protein: 5.4g**	**Carbs: 7.4g**	**Fat: 36.8g**

118. Spicy Thai Soup

Ingredients

1 3/4 lbs. boneless skinless chicken thighs

4 cups chicken broth (or stock)

1 can (14 oz) coconut milk (lite or full-fat)

1 1/2 cups white mushrooms

2 lemongrass stalks

1 small red onion

3 garlic cloves

3 inch piece ginger root

2 tablespoons pure fish sauce

1 1/2 teaspoons red curry paste

2 limes

1 jalapeño pepper

Small bunch cilantro

1 tablespoon coconut oil

Water

Directions

Thinly slice bottom 2/3 of lemongrass. Peel chop garlic and ginger. Add to medium pot with chicken broth. Heat over medium-high-heat and bring to boil. Switch to low heat and leave to simmer for about 30 minutes. Strain liquid and reserve. Heat pot over medium heat. Add coconut oil to hot pot. Roughly chop chicken and add to hot oiled pot. Sauté and brown for 5 minutes. Quarter mushrooms and add to pot. Sauté for 5 minutes. Stir in red curry paste, fish sauce, and juice of 1 lime. Add reserved chicken broth and coconut milk. Stir to combine and bring to a simmer. Switch to low heat and leave to simmer for about 20 minutes. Skim off and discard any excess fat that rises to the top. Peel and slice red onion. Add to pot and stir. Cook about 5 minutes, until onion softens. Remove from heat. Roughly chop add 1/2 to pot and stir to combine. Slice jalapeño into rings and cut lime into wedges. Transfer to serving dish. Sprinkle remaining cilantro and jalapeño slices over dish. Serve hot with lime wedges.

Serves: 4	**Prep Time: 15 mins.**	**Cooking Time: 1 hr.**
Calories: 643	**Protein: 57g**	**Carbs: 24.1g**	**Fat: 36.8g**

119. Southern Style Egg Salad

Ingredients

8 cage-free eggs
1 avocado, sliced and pitted
1 celery stalk
1/4 sweet onion
1/4 cup sweet pickle relish (or dill pickle relish + 1
tablespoon raw honey, agave or date butter)

1/4 cup organic mustard
2 teaspoons paprika
1/2 teaspoon ground black pepper
1/4 teaspoon Celtic sea salt

Directions

Add some lightly salted water on high heat and allow to boil. Leave enough room in pot for eggs. Carefully place your eggs into the boiling water then leave to cook for about 10 minutes. Drain eggs into colander in sink. Fill a second pot with cold water then add in the eggs. Allow cold water to run over eggs until they are cool. Scoop out the flesh of your avocado into medium mixing bowl. Thinly slice celery. Peel and finely dice onion. Add to mixing bowl with relish, mustard, salt and spices. Mix with large spoon to combine. Crack cooled eggs and peel off shells. Add boiled eggs to medium mixing bowl. Use a fork or knife to chop eggs. Use a large spoon to mash and mix your ingredients so that it becomes smooth with soft chunks forms. Stir to combine. Transfer to serving dish and serve immediately. Or refrigerate about 20 minutes and serve chilled.

Serves: 4	**Prep Time: 5 mins.**		**Cooking Time: 15 mins.**
Calories: 102	**Protein: 2g**	**Carbs: 7.9g**	**Fat: 8.1g**

120. Meaty Texas Chili

Ingredients

16 oz (1 lb) lean grass-fed ground beef (or elk,
bison, turkey or chicken)
15 oz (1 can) organic tomato sauce
29 oz (2 cans) organic diced tomatoes
1 cup water
1 cup cashews
1 small onion
1 bell pepper
2 cloves garlic

2 tablespoons chili powder
1 1/2 tablespoons smoked paprika (or paprika)
1 tablespoon ground cumin
1 teaspoon Mexican oregano (or dried oregano)
1 teaspoon ground black pepper
1/2 teaspoon cayenne pepper
1 teaspoon Celtic sea salt
1 tablespoon coconut oil

Directions

Heat medium pot over medium-high heat. Add 1 tablespoon coconut oil to hot pan. Peel onion and garlic. Remove stems, seeds and veins from bell pepper. Roughly chop and add to food processor or high-speed blender. Pulse until finely minced. Add minced veggies to hot skillet and sauté for about 1 minute. Add ground beef and spices. Brown beef for about 5 minutes. Stir with whisk to break up meat well, or wooden spoon to keep beef chunkier. Add whole cans of diced tomatoes and tomato sauce, and water. Stir to combine. Bring to a simmer, then reduce heat to medium and cover pot loosely with lid to prevent splatter. Simmer about 30 minutes. Stir occasionally. Remove from heat and transfer to serving dish. Use large serving spoon or ladle to serve hot.

Serves: 4	**Prep Time: 5 mins.**		**Cooking Time: 40 mins.**
Calories: 479	**Protein: 26.2g**	**Carbs: 36.2g**	**Fat: 26g**

121. Oven-Fried Chicken

Ingredients

32 oz (2 lb.) bone-in, skinless chicken
3/4 cup fine almond flour
3/4 cup almond meal (or almond flour)
2 cage free eggs
1/3 cup nut milk

1/2 teaspoon cayenne pepper
1 teaspoon ground black pepper
1 1/2 teaspoons paprika
1 1/2 tablespoons Celtic sea salt
Coconut oil (in spray bottle)

Directions

Preheat oven to 350 degrees F. Fill spray bottle with warm coconut oil. Line sheet pan with aluminum foil. Place metal cooling or baking rack over lined sheet pan. Generously spray metal rack with coconut oil to coat. Set second sheet pan aside. Add almond meal and/or flour to small mixing bowl with 1 tablespoon salt and spices.

Mix to combine with fork or whisk to break up clumps. In shallow dish, beat eggs and nut milk until combined. Use serving spoon or measuring cup to dust second sheet pan with layer of almond flour mixture onto. Sprinkle chicken with 1/2 tablespoon salt.

Dip and coat all chicken pieces in egg mixture then lay on second sheet pan, over layer of almond flour mixture. Use spoon or measuring cut to sprinkle almond flour mixture from mixing bowl over dipped chicken. Pat almond flour mixture into chicken on all sides until well coated. Transfer coasted chicken to prepared wire rack. Generously spray coated chicken with coconut oil.

Bake 60 - 70 minutes, until coating is crisp and chicken is cooked through. Switch the oven off then transfer to a cool place to cool about 10 minutes. Then place crispy chicken on paper towels to drain, if desired. Transfer to serving dish and serve immediately.

Serves: 4	Prep Time: 10 mins.		Cooking Time: 1 hr.
Calories: 354	Protein: 40.9 g	Carbs: 4g	Fat: 19.5g

122. Portobello Burger

Ingredients

4 large Portobello mushroom caps
12 oz grass-fed ground beef (or chicken, turkey, bison, elk, etc.)
1/2 white onion
Cracked black pepper, to taste
Celtic sea salt, to taste
Coconut oil (for cooking)
Portobello Cheese Sauce
4 Portobello stems

3/4 cup cashews
2 tbsp. nutritional yeast
1/2 lemon
1/4 tsp. mustard powder
1/4 tsp. white pepper
1/4 tsp. Celtic sea salt
Water
Bacon fat or coconut oil (for cooking)

Directions

Soak cashews in enough water to cover for at least 4 hours, or overnight in refrigerator. Drain and rinse. Preheat oven to 450 degrees F. Heat small pan over medium heat. Add 1 tablespoon bacon fat or coconut oil to hot pan. Line sheet pan with aluminum foil. Place metal cooling or baking rack over lined sheet pan. Remove stems from Portobello mushroom caps.

Chop and reserve stems. Place mushroom caps gill-side up on prepared sheet pan. Drizzle caps lightly with coconut oil. Peel onion and slice crosswise into 2 full 1/4 inch cross sections. Keep rings intact and place on prepared sheet pan. Drizzle slightly with coconut oil and sprinkle with salt and pepper. Form ground beef into 3/4-inch patties. Place on prepared sheet pan and sprinkle with salt and pepper.

Bake about 12 minutes, for medium-well burgers. Remove from oven and sprinkle mushroom caps with salt and pepper. For Portobello Cheese Sauce, add chopped mushrooms stems to hot oiled pan. Allow to sauté so that it becomes soft and caramelized lightly, should take about 5 minutes. Stir occasionally. Juice lemon into food processor or high-speed blender. Add cashews, nutritional yeast, salt and spices to processor. Process until smooth, about 2 minutes. Add enough water to reach desired consistency.

Add mixture to sautéed mushrooms and stir to heat Portobello Cheese Sauce through, about 2 minutes. Remove from heat. Transfer 2 mushroom caps to serving dish, gill-side up. Top with roasted onion ring slice, then hamburger patty. Spoon Portobello Cheese Sauce over patty and top with remaining Portobello caps, gill-side down. Serve hot.

Serves: 2　　　　**Prep Time: 10 mins.**　　　　**Cooking Time: 35 mins.**
Calories: 475　　　**Protein: 36 g**　　**Carbs: 13.3g**　　　**Fat: 31.3 g**

123. Mushroom Masala

Ingredients

1 head cauliflower
1 1/2 cups tomato purée (or tomato sauce)
1 pint (2 cups) mushrooms
1 onion
1 chili pepper
1 /2 green bell pepper
1 large garlic clove
1 inch piece fresh ginger

2 teaspoons coriander leaves (optional)
1 teaspoon garam masala
1/2 teaspoon cayenne pepper
1/2 teaspoon ground coriander
1/2 teaspoon Celtic sea salt
3 tablespoons bacon fat (or coconut oil or ghee)

Directions

Roughly chop cauliflower, then rice cauliflower in food processor, or mince. Add your cauli-rice into a pot with enough water to cover. Heat pot over medium heat and cook until just tender, about 8 minutes. Drain and transfer to serving dish. Heat medium pan over medium heat. Add bacon fat, oil or butter to hot pan. Peel and finely dice onions. Remove seeds, veins and stem from bell pepper and dice. Slice chili pepper. Peel and mince garlic and onion. Set your oil on to get hot then add in your onions and garlic to sauté for about 5 minutes. Slice mushrooms and add to pan with tomato, salt and spices. Add coriander to pan. Sauté and let simmer about 10 - 12 minutes, stirring occasionally. Serve and enjoy.

Serves: 8
Calories: 65

Prep Time: 10 mins.
Protein: 3.6 g

Carbs: 12.1g

Cooking Time: 25 mins.
Fat: 1.4 g

PREDIABETES BEVERAGES & SMOOTHIE RECIPES

124. Beet Coconut Water Detox

Ingredients

1 medium size raw beet, peeled and coarsely chopped

2 cups chilled unsweetened coconut water
1 lemon, juiced

Directions

Toss all your ingredients into your blender and allow to process until it becomes liquified. Garnish with a lemon slice.

Serves: 1	**Prep Time: 5 mins.**	**Cooking Time: 0 mins.**
Calories: 137	**Protein: 4.9g**	**Carbs: 28.9g**	**Fat: 1.2 g**

125. Spiced Green Tea Tonic

Ingredients

1 green teabag
¼ teaspoon turmeric
¼ teaspoon cinnamon

1 cup purified water, near boiling (green tea leaves are delicate and don't stand up well to boiling water)

Directions

Place teabag in mug and add turmeric and cinnamon. Pour in hot water and allow to steep for approximately 2 minutes. Remove the bag and stir thoroughly to dissolve the spices.

Serves: 1	**Prep Time: 10 mins.**	**Cooking Time: 0 mins.**
Calories: 4	**Protein: 0.2g**	**Carbs: 1.1g**	**Fat: 0g**

126. Whole Food Protein Shake

Ingredients

2 Tablespoons hemp seeds
2 Tablespoons chia seeds, soaked overnight
2 Tablespoons pumpkin seeds
2 Tablespoons almond butter
4 walnuts
3 Brazil nuts

1 Tablespoon coconut butter
1 banana
1 cup wild blueberries
1 cup water
1 cup unsweetened almond milk

Directions

Toss all your ingredients into your blender and allow to process until it becomes creamy and smooth.

Serves: 1	**Prep Time: 15 mins.**	**Cooking Time: 0 mins.**
Calories: 224	**Protein: 16g**	**Carbs: 11.1g**	**Fat: 62g**

127. CALL it a Smoothie

Ingredients

1 Tablespoon lemon juice
1 Tablespoon lime juice
¼ cup ice
¾ cup cucumber, peeled, cut into chunks

1 Tablespoon mashed avocado
2 pinches sea salt
2 pinches black pepper

Directions

Toss all your ingredients into your blender and allow to process until it becomes creamy and smooth.

Serves: 1   **Prep Time: 5 mins.**   **Cooking Time: 0 mins.**
Calories: 411   **Protein: 5.7g**   **Carbs: 28.7g**   **Fat: 62g**

128. Coconut Pumpkin Spiced Smoothie

Ingredients

1 frozen banana
¼ cup pureed organic pumpkin
1 cup coconut milk

2 teaspoons pumpkin pie spice
1 cup ice cubes

Directions

Toss all your ingredients into your blender and allow to process until it becomes creamy and smooth.

Serves: 2   **Prep Time: 5 mins.**   **Cooking Time: 0 mins.**
Calories: 307   **Protein: 10.4g**   **Carbs: 23.9g**   **Fat: 19.8g**

PREDIABETES SOUPS & STEW RECIPES

129. Classic Chicken Noodle Soup

Ingredients:

extra-virgin olive oil 1 tbsp.
1 cup carrots, chopped
1 cup celery, chopped
1 yellow onion, chopped
5 cups chicken broth
3 cups water
1 package of fresh poultry
herbs blend (rosemary, sage, and thyme)
Bakers twine
2 bay leaves

1 rotisserie chicken, skin removed
and meat pulled from bone
(approximately 4 cups)
½ teaspoon garlic powder
½ tsp. kosher salt
½ tsp. black pepper
14 ounces plain Udon noodles, broken into
thirds
1 cup fresh parsley, roughly chopped
2 scallions, diced

Directions:

Add your olive oil into a stock pot on medium heat. Add carrots, celery, and onions. Sauté until onions are translucent, about 5 minutes. Once vegetables start to soften, add broth and water. Lower heat to medium. Make a bundle out of poultry herbs and tie tightly with the baker's twine. Toss bundle and bay leaves into soup. Add chicken, garlic powder, salt, and pepper to soup.

Cover, raise heat to high and allow soup to reach a boil. Once soup has reached a boil, bring to a simmer and cook 5 minutes or until vegetables are tender. While soup is cooking, prepare Udon noodles according to package directions. When noodles are cooked and drained, divide them among 8 bowls. Remove soup from heat. Remove and discard herb bundle. Stir in parsley. Ladle soup over noodles and garnish with scallions. Serve immediately.

Serves: 8	Prep Time: 10 mins.		Cooking Time: 12 mins.
Calories: 170	Protein: 22g	Carbs: 11g	Fat: 4.5g

130. Slow-Cooker Fire Roasted Tomato and White Bean Soup

Ingredients:

28 oz. tomatoes, fire roasted, diced,
undrained
15 oz. cannellini beans, rinsed and drained
5 cups low sodium vegetable broth
½ cup brown rice, uncooked
¾ cup white onion, finely chopped
4 cloves garlic, minced

1 tablespoon dried basil
2 bay leaves
⅛ teaspoon crushed red pepper
¼ teaspoon salt
¼ teaspoon freshly ground black pepper
3 cups Swiss chard, chopped
½ cup shaved parmesan cheese

Directions:

Combine tomatoes, beans, broth, rice, onion, garlic, basil, bay leaves, red pepper, salt, and pepper in a 6 to 7 quart slow-cooker. Cook on low for 6 hours. Add Swiss chard and cook 15 minutes or until leaves are tender. Discard bay leaves. Serve in bowls and top with shaved parmesan cheese.

Serves: 6	Prep Time: 20 mins.		Cooking Time: 6 hrs. 15 mins.
Calories: 200	Protein: 11g	Carbs: 30g	Fat: 3g

131. Farro Minestrone Soup

Ingredients:

1 cup farro, uncooked
1 tablespoon extra-virgin olive oil
1 cup chopped yellow onion
2 cups chopped carrots
1 cup chopped celery
3 cloves of garlic, sliced
32 ounces can of diced tomatoes
(or 4 cups of chopped fresh tomatoes)

1 tablespoon dried Italian seasoning
1 teaspoon kosher salt
1 teaspoon freshly ground pepper
32 ounces of low-sodium vegetable stock
kidney beans, 15.5oz., drained and rinsed
15.5 ounce can garbanzo
(chickpeas) beans, rinsed and drained
¾ cup freshly grated parmesan cheese

Directions:

Cook Farro according to package instructions. Fluff with fork. Set aside. While farro is cooking, chop vegetables. In a large saucepan add oil, onions, carrots, celery, and garlic. Cook covered over low heat until softened, about 10 to 15 minutes, stirring occasionally. Add tomatoes, Italian seasoning, salt, pepper, and stock. Cook covered over low to medium heat for 20 minutes, stirring occasionally. Stir in kidney and garbanzo beans and Farro. Cook covered for 10 minutes. Top with parmesan cheese and serve.

Serves: 12   **Prep Time: 15 mins.**   **Cooking Time: 45 mins.**
Calories: 230   **Protein: 11g**   **Carbs: 38g**   **Fat: 4g**

132. Manhattan Clam Chowder

Ingredients:

2 tablespoons canola oil
1 cup white onion, chopped
⅛ teaspoon crushed red pepper
3 cloves garlic, minced
2 large carrots or 1 cup, chopped
3 celery stalks, chopped
1 large baking potato or 1 ½ cups, peeled and
cut in ½ inch cubes
¼ cup dry red wine

28 oz. whole peeled tomatoes, undrained
1 cup clam juice
4 cups low sodium vegetable broth
3 tablespoons tomato paste
3 bay leaves
2 teaspoons dried oregano
¼ teaspoon freshly ground black pepper
1-pound frozen clam meat, unthawed
Italian parsley, 1 cup, roughly chopped

Directions:

In a 6 to 8-quart Dutch oven or sauce pan, heat oil over medium-high heat. Add onion and crushed red pepper. Cook until onion is translucent, about 3 to 5 minutes. Add garlic, carrots, celery, and potatoes. Sauté vegetables for 5 minutes, stirring continuously. Scrape caramelized bits of onion and vegetables off pan. Add red wine. Reduce heat to medium. Using kitchen shears roughly cut apart whole peeled tomatoes (while in can).

Add tomatoes, clam juice, broth, tomato paste, bay leaves, oregano, and pepper. Cover and cook until vegetables are tender, stirring occasionally, about 25 to 30 minutes. When vegetables are tender, increase heat to medium-high heat and stir in clams. Cook 3 minutes. Remove from heat and stir. When vegetables are tender, increase heat to medium-high heat and stir in clams. Cook 3 minutes. Remove from heat and stir in fresh parsley. Serve immediately.

Serves: 6   **Prep Time: 15 mins.**   **Cooking Time: 46 mins.**
Calories: 230   **Protein: 22g**   **Carbs: 16g**   **Fat: 6g**

133. Vegetable Lentil Soup

Ingredients:

1 tablespoon extra-virgin olive oil

½ cup chopped medium yellow onion

2 celery stalks, chopped

1 ½ cup chopped carrots

3 garlic cloves, minced

1 quart low-sodium vegetable broth

1 ¼ cup lentils

15 ounces can diced tomatoes

¼ teaspoon kosher salt

½ teaspoon freshly ground pepper

1 teaspoon Italian seasoning

1 bay leaf

2 cups kale, chopped

Directions:

Heat oil in a large saucepan over medium heat, about 2 minutes. Add onions, celery, and carrots. Cook over medium heat, stirring occasionally until soft, about 8 to 10 minutes. Stir in garlic. Add broth, lentils, tomatoes, salt, pepper, Italian seasoning, and bay leaf and stir. Bring to a boil. Cover. Switch the heat to low and allow to cook for about 25 minutes or until the lentils get soft. Remove bay leaf. Add kale and stir until wilted. Serve immediately.

Serves: 6	**Prep Time: 15 mins.**	**Cooking Time: 37 mins.**
Calories: 144	**Protein: 6g**	**Carbs: 20g**	**Fat: 5g**

134. Carrot Coriander Soup

Ingredients:

1 large onion, sliced thin

2 tablespoons canola oil

1 garlic glove, minced

1 teaspoon ground coriander

10 carrots, fresh (about 1 ½ pounds), sliced thin

2 new potatoes (medium size), peeled and quartered

5 cups rich low sodium chicken broth

1 ¼ cups freshly squeezed orange juice

½ teaspoon kosher salt

½ teaspoon white pepper

¼ cup minced fresh cilantro (for garnish)

Directions:

Place onion and oil in a large stock pot. Cook over medium low heat, stirring until the onion is softened. Add garlic and cook the mixture, stirring constantly, for 2 minutes. Add coriander and cook the mixture for 2 more minutes, continuing to stir. Add the carrots and potatoes and cook the mixture, still stirring, for 2 minutes longer. Add stock, juice, salt and white pepper. Allow the liquid to boil, seal the lid, and leave to simmer. Continue to cook the mixture for 20 to 30 minutes on low heat, until the carrots are tender, stirring occasionally. Transfer the soup carefully, to a blender and puree until smooth. Pour soup into bowls. Garnish with fresh cilantro. Serve hot.

Serves: 8	**Prep Time: 15 mins.**	**Cooking Time: 36 mins.**
Calories: 143	**Protein: 4g**	**Carbs: 24g**	**Fat: 4g**

135. Moroccan Vegetable Stew

Ingredients:

Spice mixture:

2 pinches of saffron
1 teaspoon cumin
1 teaspoon ground ginger
½ teaspoon kosher salt
½ teaspoon turmeric
½ teaspoon ground cinnamon
½ teaspoon cardamom
½ teaspoon coriander
½ teaspoon ground nutmeg
½ teaspoon freshly ground
black pepper

Soup mixture:

2 tablespoons extra virgin olive oil
1 small onion, diced
3 garlic cloves, diced
3 carrots, peeled and sliced
1 small potato, peeled and sliced in quarters
½ sweet potato, peeled and sliced in quarters
1, (28 ounce) can plum tomatoes
1 cup quinoa
½ head of cauliflower, stemmed and cut into florets
1 small zucchini, sliced
1 cup canned chickpeas, rinsed and drained
2 tablespoons golden raisins

Directions:

Mix together all your spices in a bowl. Heat a 5 to 6-quart Dutch oven or large sauce pan over medium-high heat. Add spice mixture and toast until fragrant, about 1 minute. Return toasted spices to small bowl and set aside. In the same pan, heat oil over medium heat and add onions. Cook until softened, about 5 minutes. Add garlic, carrots, and potatoes. Sauté 2 to 3 minutes.

With tomatoes in can, cut into smaller pieces using kitchen shears. Add to pan. Next, stir in spices. Bring to a simmer and cook until vegetables are just tender, about 20 minutes. While vegetables are cooking, cook quinoa according to package directions. Once potatoes and carrots are just tender, add cauliflower, zucchini, and chickpeas. Cook until vegetables are tender, about 10 minutes. Stir in raisins. Serve over ⅓ cup quinoa.

Serves: 5	Prep Time: 20 mins.		Cooking Time: 40 mins.
Calories: 270	Protein: 10g	Carbs: 40g	Fat: 10g

136. Thai-Style Coconut Shrimp Soup

Ingredients:

1, (16 ounce) bag frozen shrimp (tail-on), thawed
1 teaspoon canola oil
4 cloves garlic, minced
1 tablespoon fresh ginger, minced
⅛ teaspoon crushed red pepper
4 cups low sodium vegetable broth
½ cup water
1, (13.5 ounce) can lite coconut milk
2 teaspoons oyster sauce

2 teaspoons low sodium tamari or soy sauce
1 teaspoon toasted sesame oil
7-ounce buckwheat soba noodles
2 cups shiitake mushrooms, sliced
4 heads of baby bok choy, quartered
½ cup cilantro leaves
2 scallions, diced
1 red chili pepper, sliced in wheels (seeds removed)
1 lime, cut into wedges

Directions:

Rinse and drain shrimp. Set aside. In a large Dutch oven or stock pot, heat canola oil over medium-high heat. Add garlic, ginger, and crushed red pepper. Cook until just fragrant, about 1 to 2 minutes. Add vegetable broth, water, coconut milk, sweet chili sauce, tamari, oyster sauce, and sesame oil. Bring to a boil. While broth is boiling, add soba noodles and mushrooms. Cook one minute. Add shrimp and bok choy. Cook the shrimp for about 3 minutes (the shrimp should be pink). Remove from heat and garnish with cilantro leaves, scallions, chili pepper, and lime. Serve immediately.

Serves: 4   **Prep Time: 15 mins.**   **Cooking Time: 15 mins.**
Calories: 340   **Protein: 24g**   **Carbs: 42g**   **Fat: 10g**

137. Black Bean Soup

Ingredients:

2 cups dried black beans, rinsed and drained
6 cups cold water (for soaking the beans)
2 onions, coarsely chopped
4 cloves garlic, minced
4 stalks celery, coarsely chopped
1 tbsp olive oil

4 large carrots, coarsely chopped
1 tsp dried basil
1/2 tsp dried red pepper flakes
1 tsp cumin (to taste)
8 cups chicken or vegetable broth (about)
salt and pepper, to taste

Directions:

Soak beans overnight in cold water. Drain and rinse well. Discard soaking water. Prepare vegetables. This can be done in the processor.) Heat oil in a large soup pot. Add onions, garlic and celery. Sauté for 5 or 6 minutes on medium heat, until golden. If necessary, add a little water or broth to prevent sticking. Add drained beans, carrots, seasonings and broth. Do not add salt and pepper until beans are cooked. Cover partially and simmer until beans are tender, about 2 hours, stirring occasionally. Purée part or all of the soup, if desired. If too thick, thin with water or broth. Add salt and pepper to taste.

Serves: 10   **Prep Time: 15 mins.**   **Cooking Time: 2 hrs. 6 mins.**
Calories: 188   **Protein: 14g**   **Carbs: 29g**   **Fat: 2.1g**

138. Fruit and Vegetable "Stew"

Ingredients

3/4 cup pitted prunes
3/4 cup dried apricots
1/3–1/2 cup raisins
2 lb. carrots peeled and sliced
1 sweet potato, peeled, quartered and sliced
1/2 cup honey (to taste)

14 oz (398 ml) can pineapple chunks, drained
(reserve 1/2 cup juice)
1/2 cup orange juice
salt and pepper, to taste
2 tsp pareve tub margarine
1 tsp cinnamon

Directions

Soak raisins, apricots and prunes in boiling water to cover for 1/2 hour, until plump. Drain well. While that goes set your sweet potato and carrots to cook in your boiling water until tender (about 15 minutes). Drain well. Combine reserved pineapple juice with remaining ingredients except pineapple chunks; mix gently. Place mixture in a sprayed 3-quart casserole. Cover and bake for 35 minutes at 350°F. Add your pineapple chunks and return to bake without the cover for another 15 minutes (basting often).

Serves: 10	**Prep Time: 15 mins.**	**Cooking Time: 30 mins.**
Calories: 195	**Protein: 2g**	**Carbs: 48g** **Fat: 1.1g**

139. Easy Vegetarian Chili

Ingredients:

1 tbsp olive or canola oil
2 onions, chopped
2 green and/or red peppers, chopped
3 cloves garlic, crushed
2 cups mushrooms, sliced
2 cups cooked or canned red kidney beans
2 cups cooked or canned chickpeas
1/2 cup bulgur or couscous, rinsed
28 oz (796 ml) can tomatoes (or 6 fresh tomatoes, chopped)

1 cup bottled salsa (mild or medium)
1/2 cup water
1 tsp salt (or to taste)
1 tbsp chili powder
1 tsp dried basil
1/2 tsp each pepper, oregano and cumin
1/4 tsp cayenne
1 tbsp unsweetened cocoa powder
1 tsp sugar
1 cup corn niblets, optional

Directions:

Heat oil in a large pot. Add in your garlic, peppers and onions then sauté for about 5 minutes on medium heat. Add mushrooms and sauté 4 or 5 minutes more. Add remaining ingredients except corn. Bring to a boil and simmer, covered, for 25 minutes, stirring occasionally. Stir in corn.

Serves: 10	**Prep Time: 15 mins.**	**Cooking Time: 35 mins.**
Calories: 179	**Protein: 9g**	**Carbs: 32g** **Fat: 3g**

140. Slow Cooker Thai Chicken Soup

Ingredients

curry paste (2 tbsp., red)
coconut milk (2 (12oz.) tins)
chicken stock (2 cups)
fish sauce (2 tbsp.)
peanut butter (2 tbsp.)
chicken breasts (1 ½ lb., cut into bite size pieces)

(1bell pepper (1 red, seeded and sliced into ¼ inch slices)
onion (1, thinly sliced)
fresh ginger (1 heaped tbsp., minced)
frozen peas (1 cup, thawed)
lime juice (1 tbsp.)
cilantro for garnish

Directions

Combine the curry paste, stock, fish sauce and peanut butter in a slow cooker. Place the chicken breast, red pepper, onion and ginger in the cooker and cook on high for 4 hours. Stir in the peas and coconut milk and cook for another 30 minutes. Add in your lime juice and cilantro then serve.

Serves: 6   **Prep Time: 5 mins.**   **Cook Time: 4 hrs. 30 mins.**
Calories: 374   **Protein: 41g**   **Carbs: 14g**   **Fat: 17g**

141. Creamy and Spicy Corn Soup

Ingredients

5 ears fresh sweet corn
1 medium onion, chopped
1 tsp olive oil
½ tsp salt, plus more to taste
½ a medium Yukon gold potato, chopped
vegetable stock, 2-3 cups

3 cloves garlic, minced
1 tsp cumin
1.5 tsp chili powder
A pinch of cayenne pepper
¼ tsp black pepper

Directions

Cut the corn off the cob. Sauté the onion and garlic for 5 minutes in oil in a large pot over medium heat. Add the potato and broth and then bring to a boil. Cook until your potatoes become tender (about 10 minutes). Add the corn and cook for an additional 2-3 minutes. Add the spices and then puree the soup with a blender. Serve with toppings of choice (cilantro, tomatoes, fresh corn, avocado or cheese).

Serves: 4   **Prep Time: 10 mins.**   **Cook Time: 20 mins.**
Calories: 127   **Protein: 4g**   **Carbs: 27g**   **Fat: 0g**

142. Slow Cooker Chickpea Stew with Apricots

Ingredients

2 (15oz) tins chickpeas/garbanzo beans, drained and rinsed
1 (28oz) or 2 (14.5oz) tins diced tomatoes
1 (15oz) tin vegetable broth
2 tbsp. butter
1 onion, finely chopped
3 cloves garlic, minced
¾ cup turnip, peeled and chopped
½ cup dried apricots, chopped

zest of 1 lemon
1 tsp cumin
¼ tsp ground coriander
½ tsp salt
pinch of cayenne pepper (or more to taste)
For Serving:
cilantro, chopped
lemon wedges

Directions

Add all your ingredients into a slow cooker and mix well. Allow to cook for about 4 hours using high pressure. Serve hot with fresh cilantro and lemon wedges.

Serves: 10   **Prep Time: 10 mins.**   **Cook Time: 6 hrs.**
Calories: 364   **Protein: 19g**   **Carbs: 58g**   **Fat: 0g**

143. Hearty Lentil and Vegetable Soup

Ingredients

Vegetable broth, 4 cups
1 ½ cups brown lentils
2 carrots, peeled and chopped
2 stalks celery, sliced
½ cup chopped onion
1 bay leaf

2 garlic cloves, minced
½ tsp. cumin
½ tsp. kosher or sea salt
¼ tsp. black pepper
1 ½ tbsp. olive oil

Directions

Sauté the carrots, onions and celery in the olive oil in a medium stock pot over medium high heat. Allow to cook for about 5 minutes, so that the vegetables begin to soften. Next, toss in your garlic and stir while cooking for another 30 seconds. Stir in the remaining ingredients and then simmer for 25-30 minutes, or until the lentils and vegetables are cooked.

Serves: 6   **Prep Time: 10 mins.**   **Cook Time: 35 mins.**
Calories: 240   **Protein: 15g**   **Carbs: 36g**   **Fat: 0g**

144. Slow Cooker Minestrone

Ingredients

1 small onion, diced
1 stalk celery, diced
2 carrots, peeled and sliced
1 zucchini, sliced
1 large potato, peeled and cubed
2 cups fresh or frozen green beans
1 cup fresh or frozen peas
2 cups kale, coarsely chopped

2 cups vegetable broth or water
1 (15 ounce) tin diced tomatoes, with liquid
1 (15 ounce) tin kidney beans, drained and rinsed
½ cup vegetable or tomato juice
1 tsp. kosher or sea salt
¼ tsp. ground black pepper
4 fresh basil leaves, diced
½ cup Parmigiano Reggiano or Parmesan

Directions

Combine all ingredients, except kale, basil and parmesan in a slow cooker. Allow to cook for about 6 hours using low pressure. Stir in the kale and continue to cook until wilted, about 10 minutes.
Serve garnished with the basil and cheese.

Serves: 6	Prep Time: 15 mins.	Cook Time: 6 hrs.	
Calories: 240	Protein: 8g	Carbs: 22g	Fat: 0g

145. Sausage and Red Pepper Soup

Ingredients

1 lb. regular chicken sausage
1 medium yellow onion, diced
3 large red bell peppers, diced
4 large garlic cloves, minced
10 cup low sodium chicken broth
2 cups wild rice, uncooked

1-1/2 tsp kosher salt
1 tsp dried basil
1 tsp dried thyme
1 tsp dried savory
1 tsp freshly ground black pepper
2 oz fresh spinach, chopped

Directions

Allow your sausage to brown in your skillet on medium heat. Be sure to break up the meat while it cooks so no large pieces remain. Add the onion and red pepper and cook for another 3-4 minutes. Add the garlic and sauté for another minute. Add all the ingredients, with an exception of your spinach, in a slow cooker and mix well. Allow to cook for about 8 hours with low pressure. Stir in the spinach and season to taste. Allow to cook for about 10 minutes, or until the spinach is wilted. Serve hot.

Serves: 8	Prep Time: 15 mins.	Cook Time: 8 hrs.	
Calories: 424	Protein: 21g	Carbs: 39g	Fat: 21g

146. Quinoa with Pomegranates & Butternut Squash

Ingredients

quinoa (1 cup, cooked)
butternut squash (1/2 cup, cubed and cooked)
pomegranate seeds (2 tbsp.)
orange zest (1 tbsp.)

olive oil (1 tbsp.)
orange juice (2 tbsp.)
Salt and pepper (to taste)

Directions

Combine all ingredients and mix well. Refrigerate until serving.

Serves: 2   **Prep Time: 10 mins.**   **Cook Time: 0 mins.**
Calories: 205   **Protein: 4g**   **Carbs: 28g**   **Fat: 9g**

147. Black Bean and Quinoa Chili Bowl

Ingredients

1 (15-ounce) tin black beans, drained and rinsed
1 clove garlic, minced
½ cup chopped onions
1 tbsp. chili powder
1 tsp. ground cumin
1 cup uncooked quinoa (any variety), well rinsed

Corn, 1½ cups, frozen, or drained from the can
1 red bell pepper, stemmed, seeded, and diced
1 (14.5 ounce) tin diced fire-roasted tomatoes
3 cups vegetable broth
1 tbsp. extra virgin olive oil
½ tsp. kosher or sea salt
1/8 tsp. cayenne pepper

Directions

Sauté the onion and bell pepper in olive oil over medium heat in a skillet. Next, toss in your garlic and stir while cooking for another 30 seconds, or until fragrant. Add in the stock, tomatoes and juice, quinoa, salt, chili powder, cumin and cayenne pepper. Simmer for 20 minutes on high, or until the quinoa begins to soften. Stir in the corn and black beans and cook for 5 minutes, or until cooked through. Serve hot.

Serves: 6   **Prep Time: 10 mins.**   **Cook Time: 30 mins.**
Calories: 281   **Protein: 14g**   **Carbs: 46g**   **Fat: 0g**

148. Mushroom & Quinoa Sauté

Ingredients

1 cup quinoa, rinsed
1 lb. mushrooms, sliced
1 small onion, finely diced
1 tbsp. light butter

4 cloves garlic, minced
1 tsp. dried thyme
Salt & pepper to taste

Directions

Prepare the quinoa according to package directions. Meanwhile, sauté the onion, garlic, mushroom and thyme for 5 minutes over medium high heat. Add in your quinoa then season using your salt and pepper to taste.

Serves: 4   **Prep Time: 5 mins.**   **Cook Time: 20 mins.**
Calories: 216   **Protein: 5g**   **Carbs: 35g**   **Fat: 5g**

149. Indian Vegetable Curry

Ingredients

coconut milk (1 cup, unsweetened)

cauliflower florets (3 cups, cut into bite-size pieces)

carrot (1 large, sliced 1/4-inch-thick diagonally)

yellow onion (1 medium, halved, thinly sliced lengthwise)

fresh ginger (1 tbsp., minced)

garlic (2 tsp., minced)

curry powder (2 tsp., hot)

salt

baby spinach (3 oz.)

chickpeas (1 (15-oz.), drained and rinsed)

plum tomatoes (2 medium, cut into ½" pcs)

fresh cilantro (3 tbsp., chopped)

Directions

Set a 12-inch skillet over medium-low flame, combine the coconut milk, carrot, cauliflower, ginger, garlic, onion, curry powder, and 1 tsp. salt; stir. Turn up heat to high and allow to boil. Simmer, cover, and cook, stirring frequently, until the cauliflower becomes tender, roughly 10 minutes. (If the water dissolves too quickly, stir in a quarter cup of water at intervals)

Add the chickpeas, spinach, and tomatoes, continue cooking until the chickpeas are thoroughly warmed and the spinach wilted, roughly 5 minutes. Mix in the cilantro, season to your preference with salt, and serve.

Serves: 6 **Prep Time: 5 mins.** **Cook Time: 20 mins.**

Calories: 140 **Protein: 6g** **Carbs: 18g** **Fat: 6g**

150. Burrito in a Jar

Ingredients

salsa (1 cup)

black beans (1 (15 oz.) tin, drained

cheddar cheese (1 cup, reduced fat, shredded)

Greek Yogurt (1/2 cup, non-fat)

Directions

Place a ¼ cup salsa in the bottom of 4-pint jars. Top with a ¼ cup black beans, ¼ cup cheese and 2 Tbsp. of yogurt. Serve chilled.

Serves: 4 **Prep Time: 10 mins.** **Cook Time: 0 mins.**

Calories: 196 **Protein: 18g** **Carbs: 26g** **Fat: 3g**

151. Chile Con Queso Recipe

Ingredients

1 10-ounce can, diced tomatoes, drained
½ cup diced Anaheim chilies
1 ¾ cups reduced fat shredded sharp Cheddar
1 ¼ cups skim milk
1 large onion, chopped
3 cloves garlic, minced
¼ cup fresh cilantro, chopped

¼ cup sliced green onions
2 tsp lime juice
1 tsp salt
1/8 tsp black pepper
1 tsp ground cumin
1 tsp chili powder

Directions

Sauté the onions and garlic in cooking spray over medium heat for 4-5 minutes. Add the milk and bring to a simmer. Stir in the cheese until melted. Add the remaining ingredients and cook for an additional 2-3 minutes, or until cooked through. Serve hot, garnished with additional cilantro, if desired.

Serves: 12   **Prep Time: 5 mins.**   **Cook Time: 15 mins.**
Calories: 53   **Protein: 1g**   **Carbs: 53g**   **Fat: 1g**

PREDIABETES BAKING & DESSERT RECIPES

152. Cheesy Jalapeño "Cornbread"

Ingredients

1 1/2 cups almond flour

3 cage-free eggs

1/2 cup coconut oil (or coconut or cacao butter, melted) (or sub 1/4 cup with unsweetened applesauce)

1/4 cup nutritional yeast

2 fresh jalapeños (or 1/4 cup pickled jalapeño slices)

2 tablespoons organic apple cider vinegar

2 teaspoons baking powder

1/2 teaspoon paprika

1/2 teaspoon ground turmeric or mustard (optional)

1/2 teaspoon white pepper

Directions

Preheat oven to 350 degrees F. Lightly coat baking dish or cast-iron pan with coconut oil. Beat eggs in medium mixing bowl with hand mixer or whisk until thick and slightly frothy. Add oil or butter, nutritional yeast and vinegar. Mix well. Mix in almond meal, baking powder, and spices until combined. Remove stems from fresh jalapenos. Slice and remove seeds. Stir in fresh or pickled jalapeño slices. Pour batter into prepared baking dish or pan and bake 30 -35 minutes, until edges are golden brown and top is firm. Remove from oven. Slice and serve warm. Or allow to cool to temperature and serve.

Serves: 12	Prep Time: 5 mins.		Cooking Time: 25 mins.
Calories: 97	Protein: 4.2g	Carbs: 2.6g	Fat: 7.8g

153. Basic Banana Bread

Ingredients

1 cup almond flour

1/4 cup coconut flour

2 overripe bananas

2 cage-free eggs

1/4 cup raw honey (or agave, date butter or stevia)

1/4 cup coconut oil (or coconut or cacao butter, melted) (or unsweetened applesauce or nut butter)

1 tablespoon baking powder

2 teaspoons ground cinnamon

1/2 teaspoon ground nutmeg

1 teaspoon vanilla

1/2 teaspoon Celtic sea salt

Directions

Preheat oven to 350 degrees F. Coat small or medium loaf pan with coconut oil. Peel bananas and add to medium mixing bowl. Beat with hand mixer or whisk. Add eggs, oil or butter, and sweetener. Beat well, about 1 - 2 minutes. In separate bowl, blend flours, baking powder, salt and spices. Combine your banana mixture and flour mixture together then transfer to a prepared loaf pan and bake for about 35 minutes, or until browned and firm in the center. Remove from oven and set aside to cool. Slice and serve warm.

Serves: 8	Prep Time: 5 mins.		Cooking Time: 40 mins.
Calories: 108	Protein: 2.8g	Carbs: 17.4g	Fat: 3.6g

154. Gingerbread Cookies

Ingredients

1 cup almond flour
2 cage-free eggs
1/2 cup dried pitted dates
1/4 cup raw honey (or dark agave)
1/4 cup coconut oil (or cacao butter, melted)
1/2 teaspoon baking soda
1/2 teaspoon baking powder
2 teaspoons ground ginger

1 teaspoon ground cinnamon
1 teaspoon vanilla
1/2 teaspoon ground cloves
1/2 teaspoon ground black pepper
1/4 teaspoon Celtic sea salt
Natural sarsaparilla or root beer beverage, or nut milk (optional)

Directions

Preheat oven to 350 degrees F. Line sheet pan with parchment or baking mat. Add dates, honey or agave and eggs to food processor or high-speed blender. Process until thick smooth mixture forms, about 2 minutes. Add almond flour, oil or butter, baking soda and powder, salt and spices to processor. Process until thick mixture comes together, about 1 minute. Add sarsaparilla, root beer or nut milk to thin as necessary. Batter should resemble thick cookie dough. From rounds and place on prepares sheet pan. Flatten into disks. Bake 10 - 15 minutes, until browned around edges and cooked through, but still soft. Remove from oven and let cool at about 10 minutes. Transfer to serving dish and serve warm. Or cool completely and serve room temperature.

Serves: 12   **Prep Time: 5 mins.**   **Cooking Time: 15 mins.**
Calories: 121   **Protein: 1.7g**   **Carbs: 15.5g**   **Fat: 6.2g**

155. Strawberry Toaster Pastry

Ingredients

Crust
2 cups almond flour
2 cage-free eggs
1/4 cup coconut oil (or ghee, cacao butter or coconut butter, softened)
1 tablespoon date butter (or honey or agave)
1/4 teaspoon baking soda
1/4 teaspoon vanilla

1/2 teaspoon Celtic sea salt

Filling
2 cups chopped strawberries (about 3/4 pint whole strawberries) (fresh or frozen)
2 tablespoons raw honey (or agave)
1/2 teaspoon vanilla
1/4 teaspoon Celtic sea salt

Directions

Preheat oven to 400 degrees. Line sheet pan with parchment or baking mat. Cover cutting board with parchment. For Crust, sift almond flour into medium mixing bowl. Add baking soda, vanilla and salt. In a small mixing bowl, whisk eggs and date butter. Add flour mixture and mix to combine. Add oil, ghee or butter and mix until malleable dough comes together.

Roll in plastic wrap or wrap tightly in parchment and refrigerate for 15 minutes. Heat medium pan over medium heat. Chop strawberries and add to hot pan with honey, vanilla and salt. Cook strawberries down until juices thicken and reduce, about 10 minutes. Stir occasionally. Remove dough from refrigerator. Roll out dough on parchment covered cutting board to about 1/8-inch-thick rectangle with rolling pin.

Use sharp knife or pizza cutter to cut dough into 4 rectangles. Scoop equal portions of Filling into center of one side of each dough rectangle. Fold bare half of dough over filled half. Press edges together, letting any trapped air escape. Crimp edges of dough together with fork. Repeat with remaining dough. Arrange pastries on prepared sheet pan and bake 15 - 20 minutes, or until golden and cooked through. Switch the oven off and serve.

Serves: 4   Prep Time: 25 mins.   Cooking Time: 20 mins.
Calories: 268   Protein: 5.2g   Carbs: 14.9g   Fat: 21.8g

156. Cocoa Zucchini Muffin

Ingredients

1 1/2 cups almond flour
2 cage-free eggs
1 small zucchini (about 1 cup grated)
1/2 cup unsweetened applesauce
1/4 cup date butter (or agave or raw honey)
1/4 cup coconut oil (or cacao or coconut butter, melted)
1/4 cup cocoa powder

2 tablespoons ground chia seed (or flax meal)
1 teaspoon baking soda
1 teaspoon baking powder
1 teaspoon vanilla
1 teaspoon ground cinnamon
1 teaspoon ground black pepper
1/2 teaspoon Celtic sea salt
1/4 cup cocoa nibs or chocolate chips (optional)

Directions

Preheat oven to 350 degrees F. Line muffin pan with paper liners or lightly coat with coconut oil. Add eggs, oil or melted butter, applesauce and date butter to food processor or high-speed blender. Process until thick, light mixture forms, about 1 - 2 minutes. Sift almond flour, cocoa powder, chia or flax meal, baking soda and powder, salt and spices into processor. Process to combine, about 1 minute. Grate zucchini and stir in with cocoa nibs or chocolate chips (optional). Use scoop or tablespoon to pour batter into prepared muffin pan. Bake for about 15 - 20 minutes, until toothpick inserted into center comes out clean. Switch the oven off and place your food to cool for about 5 minutes. Serve warm.

Serves: 12	Prep Time: 10 mins.		Cooking Time: 15 mins.
Calories: 105	Protein: 2.2g	Carbs: 3.4g	Fat: 9.8g

157. Poppy Seed Pretzel

Ingredients

1 cup coconut flour
1/2 cup tapioca flour
1/2 cup coconut oil (or cacao or coconut butter)
1/2 cup water
1 cage-free egg
2 tablespoons apple cider vinegar

1/2 teaspoon baking soda
1/2 teaspoon baking powder
Topping
1 tablespoon coconut oil (or full-fat coconut milk)
1 - 2 tablespoons poppy seeds

Directions

Preheat oven to 350 degrees F. Heat medium pan over medium-high heat. Line sheet pan with parchment or baking mat. Add oil or butter, water, vinegar and salt to pot. Bring to a boil and remove from heat. Whisk in tapioca flour. Stir until mixture congeals and comes together. Stir in baking soda and baking powder. Continue mixing for a minute. Mixture will foam and expand. Let mixture sit and cool about 5 minutes. Sift in coconut flour. Mix partially, then beat in egg.

Blend until combined. Excess coconut flour may sit in bottom of bowl. Turn out dough onto cutting board dusted with any excess coconut flour from mixture. Knead dough for 2 minutes. Cut dough into 4 equal portions. Roll out pieces into ropes and twist to form classic pretzel twist. Pinch together any crumbled dough. Arrange pretzels on lined sheet pan. For Topping, brush with coconut oil or milk and sprinkle generously with poppy seeds. Place sheet pan in oven and bake about 25 minutes, until golden cooked through. Serve warm. Or allow to cool and serve room temperature.

Serves: 4	Prep Time: 15 mins.		Cooking Time: 20 mins.
Calories: 395	Protein: 3.3g	Carbs: 20.3g	Fat: 34.6g

158. Tender Stevia Cookies

Ingredients:

2 cups whole wheat or light baking flour
¼ teaspoon salt
¾ teaspoon baking soda
1 teaspoon cinnamon
¼ cup butter, softened

1 cup stevia
1 egg, lightly beaten
½ cup buttermilk
frosting

Directions:

Heat oven to 350 degrees. In a bowl, combine your cinnamon, baking soda, salt and flour; set aside. In another bowl, beat stevia and butter together until fluffy; add egg and milk; continue beating until smooth. Stir flour mixture into egg mixture, stirring just until well blended. Spoon onto a lightly greased baking sheet, about 2-inches apart then set to bake for about 10 minutes at 350 degree oven for 10 minutes, or until lightly browned. Lightly spread cooled cookies with frosting.

Serves: 24   Prep Time: 15 mins.   Cook Time: 20 mins.
Calories: 73   Protein: 1g   Carbs: 5g   Fat: 5g

159. Tomato Juice Cake

Ingredients:

1¼ cups whole wheat or light baking flour
½ teaspoon baking soda
2 teaspoons baking powder
½ teaspoon salt
1 teaspoon cinnamon
¼ teaspoon cloves
¼ teaspoon nutmeg
½ teaspoon allspice

⅓ cup butter, softened
¼ cup applesauce
¾ cup stevia
2 large eggs
1 cup tomato juice
½ cup golden raisins (optional)
½ cups walnuts, finely ground (optional)
cream cheese frosting

Direction:

Heat oven to 350 degrees and lightly grease a baking dish. In a medium bowl, combine spices, salt, baking powder, flour and baking soda; set aside. In another bowl, beat stevia, applesauce and butter until fluffy. Add eggs individually and continue to beat until incorporated.

Add flour mixture alternately with tomato juice and beat until blended; fold in raisins and ground walnuts if desired.

Pour batter into your baking dish and set to bake for about 25 minutes, or until it passes a cake toothpick test. Cool; frost and enjoy.

Serves: 12-15   Prep Time: 15 mins.   Cook Time: 30 mins.
Calories: 157.5   Protein: 1.8g   Carbs: 30.9g   Fat: 3.4g

160. Cheesy Chive Muffins

Ingredients:

2 cups all-purpose or light baking flour
1 teaspoon salt
3 teaspoons baking powder
½ teaspoon paprika
2 eggs, lightly beaten
1 cup buttermilk

¾ cup milk
½ cup cheddar cheese, shredded
½ cup Parmesan cheese, grated
½ cup vegetable oil
3 tablespoons chives, finely chopped

Directions:

Heat oven to 350 degrees and lightly grease your muffin tin. In a large bowl, mix flour, salt, baking powder and paprika; set aside. In a medium bowl, add eggs, buttermilk, milk, cheddar cheese, Parmesan cheese and oil; mix well. Pour egg mixture into flour mixture, stirring just until the dry ingredients are moistened and a few lumps remain; stir in chives. Spoon into muffin tin then set to bake for about 15 minutes, or until a toothpick can be inserted in the center and come out clean.

Serves: 12   **Prep Time: 15 mins.**   **Cook Time: 20 mins.**
Calories: 176.7   **Protein: 6.6g**   **Carbs: 19.4g**   **Fat: 6.6g**

161. Walnut Cake

Ingredients:

3½ cups whole wheat flour
¼ teaspoon baking powder
2 teaspoons baking soda
½ cup stevia
4 large eggs
1½ cups buttermilk

½ cup butter, softened
1 teaspoon vanilla
½ teaspoon salt
1½ cups walnuts, finely ground
½ cup vegetable oil
frosting

Directions:

Heat oven to 350 degrees and lightly grease a baking dish. In a bowl, combine salt, baking powder, flour and baking soda; set aside. In another bowl, beat butter, oil and stevia together until smooth; beat in eggs individually, then vanilla. Add flour mixture to egg mixture alternately with buttermilk, beating just until smooth and blended fold in ground walnuts. Pour batter into your baking dish and set to bake for about 35 minutes, or until toothpick can be inserted in the center and come out clean. Cool; frost.

Serves: 12-15   **Prep Time: 15 mins.**   **Cook Time: 40 mins.**
Calories: 180   **Protein: 2g**   **Carbs: 28g**   **Fat: 7g**

162. Yogurt Spice Bundt Cake

Ingredients:

2 cups all-purpose or light baking flour
1 teaspoon cinnamon
1 teaspoon allspice
½ teaspoon nutmeg
½ teaspoon salt
1½ teaspoons baking soda

1¼ cups stevia
1 cup butter, softened
3 eggs
1 cup plain or vanilla yogurt
1 teaspoon vanilla
powdered stevia or frosting

Directions:

Heat oven to 325 degrees and lightly grease a Bundt pan. In a bowl, combine baking soda, salt, nutmeg, allspice, cinnamon and flour. In another bowl, beat stevia and butter together. Add eggs individually; add yogurt, vanilla, and flour mixture, beating just until blended. Pour batter into your prepared pan; set to bake for 45 minutes, or until a toothpick can be inserted in the center of the cake and come out clean. Cool; turn pan upside down over a cake plate to remove cake. Dust top with powdered stevia or frost.

Serves: 12-15	Prep Time: 15 mins.	Cook Time: 50 mins.	
Calories: 350	Protein: 4g	Carbs: 56g	Fat: 13g

163. Buttermilk Prune Muffins

Ingredients:

2 cups water
1 cup prune bits
5 tablespoons butter, softened
3 tablespoons stevia
2 eggs, lightly beaten
1 cup buttermilk, room temperature
½ teaspoon salt

½ teaspoon lemon peel powder
½ teaspoon cinnamon
¾ cup whole wheat flour
1¼ cup all-purpose or light baking flour
1 tablespoon baking powder
½ teaspoon baking soda

Directions:

Heat oven to 400 degrees. In a small saucepan, boil water; remove from heat. Add prunes and let soak for 8 minutes. Drain prunes; sift some of the flour over the prune bits; toss to coat, then set aside. In a large bowl, cream butter and stevia; add eggs and buttermilk. Add salt, lemon powder, cinnamon, flours, baking powder and baking soda, mixing just until the dry ingredients are moistened and a few lumps remain; fold in prunes. Spoon batter into greased muffin cups; bake at 400 degrees for 18 minutes, or until toothpick inserted in center comes out clean.

Serves: 12	Prep Time: 15 mins.	Cook Time: 30 mins.	
Calories: 194.9	Protein: 3.8g	Carbs: 121.2g	Fat: 3.8g

164. Bohemian Apple Kolaches

Ingredients:

2 packages active dry yeast
½ cup plus 1 tablespoon stevia
¼ cup lukewarm water
1¼ cups butter, divided, melted
2 cups milk
2 whole eggs plus 4 yolks
1 ½ teaspoons salt

½ teaspoon powdered lemon peel
1 teaspoon vanilla
6 – 7 cups whole wheat flour
Apple Filling
2 cups applesauce
1 egg, beaten, reserved
cinnamon and stevia mixed

Directions:

Heat oven to 400 degrees. Dissolve yeast in ¼ cup lukewarm water; add 1 tablespoon stevia, stir. Rest yeast mixture for 5 minutes or until bubbly. Meanwhile, combine 1 cup melted butter and milk in the microwave or a saucepan until warmed (not scalding). In a large bowl, add whole eggs and yolks plus remaining stevia and beat until thickened. Add milk and butter mixture to egg mixture; beat in salt, lemon peel and vanilla. Beat in flour, one cup at a time, until it becomes too thick to beat.

Place dough on floured pastry board and knead until smooth, about 5 minutes. Place in greased bowl, rounding up with greased side up. Cover your pastry with a towel and place it in a warm place so it can rise until doubled. Punch down dough; place on a lightly floured board and divide into 6 large pieces. Next cut each of the large pieces into 12 smaller pieces; form each into balls. Place balls on a baking sheet and brush each with melted butter; cover and let rise again until double. Press the center of each down, making a flat indentation in the center, and fill each with 1 tablespoon applesauce; let rise again, about 30 minutes. Set to bake for about 10 minutes at 400 degrees The edges should be lightly brown. Top with cinnamon stevia.

Serves: 6	Prep Time: 15 mins.	Cook Time: 1 hr. 40 mins.	
Calories: 60.6	Protein: 0.7g	Carbs: 5g	Fat: 4.2g

165. Blueberry Muffins

Ingredients:

1¾ cups all-purpose or light baking flour
⅓ cup stevia
2½ teaspoons baking powder
½ teaspoon salt

¾ cup milk
1 egg, lightly beaten
⅓ cup butter, softened
1 cup blueberries, fresh or frozen

Directions

Heat oven to 400 degrees. In a medium bowl, combine flour, stevia, baking powder and salt then set aside. In a large bowl, beat butter and stevia until creamy; add egg and milk. Add flour mixture to butter mixture and stir until the dry ingredients are moistened and a few lumps remain; fold in blueberries. Spoon batter into twelve greased muffin cups; bake at 400 degrees for 18 minutes, or until it passes a cake toothpick test. Enjoy.

Serves: 12	**Prep Time: 15 mins.**	**Cook Time: 20 mins.**
Calories: 162.8	**Protein: 7.5g**	**Carbs: 11.2g** **Fat: 3.4g**

166. Banana Pineapple Bread

Ingredients:

2 cups whole wheat flour
Baking soda, 1 tsp.
2 teaspoons baking powder
½ teaspoon salt
⅓ cup butter, softened
¼ cup applesauce

¼ cup granulated stevia
¼ cup brown stevia
2 eggs
1 cup banana, mashed
Pineapple, canned, 8oz, crushed, undrained

Directions:

Heat oven to 350 degrees. In a bowl, combine baking powder, salt and flour; set aside. Cream together butter, applesauce, and stevia; add eggs and mix well. Add flour mixture to egg mixture, stirring just until the dry ingredients are moistened and a few lumps remain; fold in mashed banana and pineapple in juice. Pour into a greased 9x5-inch loaf pan. Bake in prepared oven for about 60 minutes, or until done.

Serves: 8	**Prep Time: 15 mins.**	**Cook Time: 1 hr. 10 mins.**
Calories: 194.9	**Protein: 3.8g**	**Carbs: 121.2g** **Fat: 3.8g**

167. Tapioca Pudding

Ingredients:

4 cups milk

⅓ cup tapioca

3 eggs

1 cup stevia

1 teaspoon vanilla

whipped cream (optional)

Directions:

In a medium saucepan, heat milk until near boiling; reduce heat and add tapioca, cook on low heat for 20 minutes, or until tapioca is translucent. Stir occasionally. In a small bowl, beat eggs, stevia and vanilla together; slowly add egg mixture to saucepan; continue cooking over low heat and stirring constantly until pudding thickens to desired consistency. Refrigerate to chill. Top each serving with whipped cream if desired.

Serves: 6	**Prep Time: 15 mins.**	**Cook Time: 1 hr. 30 mins.**
Calories: 140	**Protein: 3.1g**	**Carbs: 24g** **Fat: 4g**

168. Pre-Diabetes Granola

Ingredients:

Canola oil (1/4 cup)

Honey (4 tbsp.)

Vanilla (1 ½ tsp.)

Old fashioned rolled oats (6 cups)

Almond (1 cup, slivered)

Unsweetened coconut (1/2 cup shredded)

Bran flakes (2 cups)

Walnuts (3/4 cup, chopped)

Raisins (1 cup)

Cooking spray (parchment paper can also be used)

Directions:

Prepare oven to preheat at 325 degrees F. In a saucepan cook oil and vanilla gently over low flame, occasionally stirring for roughly 5 mins. Place all (except raisins) ingredients remaining, in a large bowl and combine. Stir in honey and oil mixture slowly and ensure that all grains are properly coated.

Cover a baking tray with parchment paper or use cooking spray to spray it lightly. Spread cereal evenly in the tray and bake for 25 mins. (occasionally stirring to keep mixture from burning), or until very lightly browned, or the grains crisp. When finished, remove cereal and put to cool. Add the cup of raisins and mix well so that raisins are thoroughly spread through the grain mixture.

Serves: 10	**Prep Time: 15 mins.**	**Cook Time: 40 mins.**
Calories: 458	**Protein: 12.1g**	**Carbs: 62g** **Fat: 2.1g**

169. Vanilla Bean Shortbread Cookies

Ingredients

1 2/3 cups almond flour
2/3 cup almonds (blanched, skinless)
1/4 cup coconut oil (or cacao butter or coconut butter, melted)

1/4 cup date butter (or raw honey or agave)
1 Madagascar whole vanilla bean
1/4 teaspoon baking soda
1/4 teaspoon Celtic sea salt (plus extra)

Directions

Preheat oven to 300 degrees F. Line sheet pan with parchment or baking mat. Add almonds to food processor or high-speed blender and process until finely ground, about 2 minutes. Add ground almonds to medium mixing bowl. Sift in almond flour, baking soda and salt. Split vanilla bean pod in half and scrap insides into small mixing bowl. Add oil or melted butter and date butter. Mix to combine. Pour vanilla mixture into flour mixture and mix to form dough. Use mini ice cream scoop or tablespoon to drop portions of dough onto prepared sheet pan. Bake for 20 minutes, or until lightly browned. Switch off the oven and allow to cool for at least 5 minutes. Serve warm.

Serves: 12   **Prep Time: 5 mins.**   **Cook Time: 20 mins.**
Calories: 76   **Protein: 0.1g**   **Carbs: 0.1g**   **Fat: 8.5g**

170. Berry Cobbler

Ingredients

1 cup blueberries
1 cup raspberries
1 cup strawberries (chopped)
1 cup blackberries
2 tablespoons tapioca flour (or arrowroot powder)
1 teaspoon vanilla
1/2 teaspoon ground ginger
1/4 teaspoon Celtic sea salt
Crumble

1 cup almond flour
1/2 cup almonds
1/4 cup coconut oil (or cacao butter)
1/4 cup almond butter
1/4 cup dried pitted dates
1 teaspoon vanilla
1/2 teaspoon ground cinnamon
1/2 teaspoon Celtic sea salt
Raw honey (or agave or date butter) (optional)

Directions

Preheat oven to 350 degrees F. Lightly coat sides of baking dish with coconut oil. Add berries, vanilla, ginger and salt to medium mixing bowl. Sift tapioca into bowl and gently toss. Transfer to prepared baking dish and set aside. For Crumble, add dates, oil or butter, and almonds to food processor or high-speed blender. Pulse until dates and almonds are finely chopped or coarsely ground. Transfer to clean medium mixing bowl with almond flour, almond butter, vanilla, cinnamon and salt. Mix with hands or wooden spoon until crumbly mixture resembling moist graham cracker crust forms. Add sweetener to reach desired consistency, if necessary. Sprinkle crumble evenly over berries and bake about 25 minutes, until crumble is golden brown and crisp. Switch the oven off and allow to cool for about 5 minutes. Serve warm.

Serves: 8   **Prep Time: 5 mins.**   **Cook Time: 25 mins.**
Calories: 229   **Protein: 1.3g**   **Carbs: 29.3g**   **Fat: 13g**

171. Vanilla Peach Cake

Ingredients

4 ripe peaches
3/4 cup coconut flour
10 cage-free eggs
1/2 cup coconut oil (or cacao or coconut butter)
1/3 cup raw honey (or agave, date butter or stevia)

2 tablespoons tapioca flour (or arrowroot powder)
1 teaspoon baking soda
1 1/2 teaspoons vanilla
1 teaspoon Celtic sea salt

Directions

Preheat oven to 350 degrees F. Line square or rectangular baking dish with parchment paper, or coat with coconut oil. Slice peaches in half, twist to release from pit and remove pit. Dice 2 peaches and set aside. Roughly chop remaining peaches and add to food processor or high-speed blender. Process until almost smooth, about 1 minute. Add eggs, oil or butter, and flour to processor in 2 batches.

Continue to process for about 2 minutes so that everything gets combined, about 1 - 2 minutes. Add sweetener, baking soda, vanilla and salt. Process until light, thick batter forms. Stir in diced peaches. Transfer your batter to a baking pan and bake about 50 minutes, until it passes a cake toothpick test. Switch the oven off and allow to cool about 10 minutes. Slice and serve warm. Or let cool completely and serve room temperature or warm.

Serves: 12	**Prep Time: 10 mins.**	**Cook Time: 50 mins.**
Calories: 117	**Protein: 0.1g**	**Carbs: 9.7g** **Fat: 9.1g**

172. Cranberry Almond Cookies

Ingredients

1 1/2 cups almond flour
1 cage-free egg
1/4 cup coconut oil (or cacao or coconut butter)
1/4 cup raw honey (or agave or date butter)
1/4 cup almond butter

1/4 cup almonds
1/4 cup dried cranberries
1/2 teaspoon baking powder
1 teaspoon vanilla
1/4 teaspoon Celtic sea salt

Directions

Preheat oven to 350 degrees F. Line sheet pan with parchment or baking mat. Sift flour, baking powder and salt into medium mixing bowl. Beat with whisk or hand mixer to lighten. Add egg, oil or butter, sweetener, almond butter, vanilla and salt. Mix well to form dough. Chop almonds and add to bowl with cranberries. Mix to combine. Shape dough into 12 balls and place on prepared baking sheet. Flatten slightly with hand or spatula. Place in oven and bake 10 - 15 minutes, until golden brown along edges. Remove from oven and let cool 5 minutes. Serve warm. Or transfer to wire rack to cool completely and serve room temperature.

Serves: 12	**Prep Time: 10 mins.**	**Cook Time: 15 mins.**
Calories: 110	**Protein: 0.9g**	**Carbs: 6.7g** **Fat: 9.3g**

173. Mocha Brownie Bites

Ingredients

4 cage-free eggs
1 cup cocoa powder
1/4 cup coconut oil
1/4 cup full-fat coconut milk

1/4 cup stevia, raw honey or agave nectar
2 teaspoons instant espresso (or instant coffee)
1 teaspoon vanilla

Directions

Preheat oven to 350 degrees F. Lightly oil square baking dish or line with parchment. Add eggs, coconut oil, coconut milk and sweetener to medium mixing bowl and beat with hand mixer or whisk. Sift in cocoa powder, espresso and vanilla. Beat until well combined. Pour batter into prepared baking pan and allow to bake for about 25 minutes, until set. Allow to cool completely. Slice and serve room temperature. Or refrigerate and serve chilled.

| Serves: 16 | Prep Time: 5 mins. | | Cook Time: 25 mins. |
| Calories: 99 | Protein: 3.3g | Carbs: 8g | Fat: 7.4g |

174. Double Pumpkin Muffins

Ingredients

1 3/4 cups coconut flour
2 cage-free eggs
15 oz (1 can) organic pumpkin puree
1 cup unsweetened applesauce
1/2 cup coconut oil
1/4 cup raw/natural sweetener

2 teaspoons baking soda
1 1/2 tablespoon ground cinnamon
1/2 teaspoon ground nutmeg
1 teaspoon sea salt
1/2 cup pumpkin seeds

Directions

Preheat oven to 350 degrees F. Line muffin pan with paper liner or coat with coconut oil.
Process eggs, coconut oil, applesauce and sweetener in food processor or blender until thick and light, about 2 minutes. Pour egg mixture into medium mixing bowl. Add pumpkin puree, salt and spices and mix with hand mixer or whisk. Sift in coconut flour and baking soda. Mix until well combined. Stir in half of pumpkin seeds.
Pour batter into prepared muffin pan and sprinkle remaining pumpkin seeds over batter.
Place in oven and set to bake for about 25 minutes, so that your edges are golden.
Switch off the oven and set to cool for about 5 minutes. Serve warm.

| Serves: 12 | Prep Time: 5 mins. | | Cook Time: 25 mins. |
| Calories: 318 | Protein: 9.9g | Carbs: 27.9g | Fat: 20.1g |

175. Cinnamon Raisin Bread

Ingredients

3/4 cup coconut flour
3/4 cup almond flour
1/4 cup ground chia seed (or flax meal)
2 cage-free eggs
1/2 cup raisins
1/2 cup coconut oil

1/2 cup unsweetened applesauce
1/4 cup stevia, raw honey or agave nectar
2 tablespoons ground cinnamon
1 teaspoon baking powder
1 teaspoon sea salt
1/2 teaspoon ground black pepper (optional)

Directions

Preheat oven to 350 degrees F. Line baking pan with parchment or coat with coconut oil. In large bowl, whisk eggs with hand mixer or whisk until frothy and light. Add coconut oil, sweetener and applesauce. Blend until combined. Sift coconut and almond flour, chia meal, baking powder, salt and spices into wet ingredients. Beat until smooth and well combined. Stir in raisins. Pour batter into prepared baking pan. Set to bake for about 25 minutes, your edges should be golden. Switch the oven off and allow to cool for about 5 minutes. Slice and serve warm.

Serves: 12	**Prep Time: 5 mins.**	**Cook Time: 20 mins.**
Calories: 133	**Protein: 1.7g**	**Carbs: 8.9g** **Fat: 10.8g**

176. All-Purpose Pizza Crust

Ingredients

1/3 cup coconut flour
3 cage-free eggs
1/2 cup coconut milk
2 tablespoons flax meal (or ground chia seed)

2 tablespoons tapioca flour
1 teaspoon baking powder
1/2 teaspoon sea salt

Directions

Preheat oven to 350 degrees F. Line sheet pan with parchment paper or baking mat, or coat lightly with coconut oil. In medium bowl, beat eggs and coconut milk with hand mixer or whisk until well combined. Sift coconut and tapioca flour, flax meal, baking powder and salt into egg mixture. Beat into thick batter. Spread batter into desired shape on sheet pan with ladle or spatula. Place in oven and bake for 10 minutes, or until firm enough to flip. Carefully remove par baked crust. Peel away from sheet pan and turn over. Return crust to oven and bake for additional 8 - 10 minutes, or until cooked through. Remove crust and evenly spread with desired sauce and sprinkle with favorite toppings. Set oven to broil. Broil pizza for 1 - 2 minutes, just to heat toppings. Remove pizza and slice with knife or pizza cutter. Serve hot.

Serves: 2	**Prep Time: 5 mins.**	**Cook Time: 20 mins.**
Calories: 283	**Protein: 16g**	**Carbs: 15.8g** **Fat: 16.8g**

177. Avocado Club Muffin

Ingredients

1 cup almond flour
2 cage-free eggs
1 avocado

4 slices nitrate-free bacon
1 tablespoon stevia, raw honey or agave nectar

Directions

Preheat oven to 350 degrees F. Line muffin pan with paper liners or light coat with coconut oil. Heat medium pan over medium-high heat. Finely chop bacon and add to hot pan. Sauté until crisp and cooked through, about 5 minutes. Set aside. Beat eggs, sweetener and vinegar in medium mixing bowl with hand mixer or whisk until thick and slightly foamy. Slice avocado in half. Scoop flesh of one half into egg mixture. Add bacon and drippings, almond flour, baking powder and black pepper and mix until combined. Dice remaining avocado flesh and fold into batter. Use ice cream scoop or tablespoon to scoop your batter into your muffin pan. Set to bake for about 20 minutes, your edges should be golden brown. Switch the oven off and allow to cool for about 5 minutes. Serve warm.

Serves: 12	Prep Time: 10 mins.	Cook Time: 15 mins.	
Calories: 90	Protein: 2.9g	Carbs: 3.1g	Fat: 7.5g

178. Carrot Cake Cookie Bars

Ingredients

2 cups almond meal
2 cups shredded carrots (about 4 large carrots)
3 cage-free eggs
1/4 cup coconut oil
1/2 cup unsweetened applesauce
1/2 cup flaked coconut

1/4 cup stevia, raw honey or agave nectar
2 teaspoons vanilla
2 teaspoons ground cinnamon
1 teaspoon ground nutmeg
1/2 teaspoon ground black pepper
1/2 teaspoon sea salt

Directions

Preheat oven to 350 Degrees F. Line baking pan with parchment or coat lightly with coconut oil. Grate carrots, or process in food processor or bullet blender until finely chopped. Add to medium bowl. Add eggs, oil, applesauce and sweetener to food processor or bullet blender. Process until thickened and light, about 1 - 2 minutes. Pour egg mixture into carrots. Sift in almond flour and salt. Add vanilla and spices. Mix well with a wooden spoon or hand mixer. Stir in coconut. Press dough evenly into prepared baking pan and bake about 25 minutes, or until firm and golden brown. Switch off the oven and set to cool about 10 minutes. Slice into bars and serve warm.

Serves: 12	Prep Time: 10 mins.	Cook Time: 25 mins.	
Calories: 112	Protein: 2.6g	Carbs: 10g	Fat: 7.2g

179. Orange Cranberry Muffins

Ingredients

1 1/2 cups almond flour
2 cage-free eggs
Oranges, 2, juiced
1/4 cup coconut oil
1/4 cup dried cranberries

1 tablespoon orange zest
1 teaspoon baking powder
1/2 teaspoon vanilla
1/2 teaspoon sea salt

Directions

Preheat oven to 350 degrees F. Line muffin pan with paper liners or coconut oil. In medium bowl, beat eggs with hand mixer or whisk until light and a foamy. Add coconut oil, orange juice and zest. Beat well. Sift in almond flour, baking powder, vanilla and salt. Mix until combined. Stir in cranberries. Use ice cream scoop or tablespoon to scoop batter into prepared muffin pan. Set to bake for 20 minutes, or until it passes a cake toothpick test. Switch the oven off and serve warm.

Serves: 12	Prep Time: 5 mins.	Cook Time: 20 mins.	
Calories: 71	Protein: 1.6g	Carbs: 2.3g	Fat: 6.2g

180. Onion Crumpets

Ingredients

1/3 cup coconut flour
4 eggs
1/4 cup nut milk
2 tablespoons coconut oil
1 tablespoon unsweetened applesauce

1/2 teaspoon baking soda
1 teaspoon organic apple cider vinegar
1 teaspoon onion powder
1/4 teaspoon sea salt
1 teaspoon dehydrated onion flakes (optional)

Directions

Preheat oven to 400 degrees F. Coat 4 mini-round cake pans or 4-inch diameter ramekins with coconut oil. In small mixing bowl, mix baking soda and apple cider vinegar. Set aside and allow to froth. In medium bowl, beat eggs with hand mixer or whisk until thick and lightened. Add flour, nut milk, applesauce, onion powder and salt. Mix to combine. Add baking soda and vinegar mixture to medium bowl. Blend well until smooth. Pour batter into prepared pans or ramekins and sprinkle on dehydrated onion flakes (optional). Bake for 12 - 15 minutes, until slightly golden and center is firm to the touch. Remove muffins from oven. Loosen from sides of pans or ramekins with knife, then turn out. Serve warm. Or let cool complete and serve room temperature.

Serves: 4	Prep Time: 5 mins.	Cook Time: 15 mins.	
Calories: 206	Protein: 9.7g	Carbs: 3.8g	Fat: 17g

181. Spinach Mushroom Muffins

Ingredients

1 cup almond flour
2 eggs
1 cup fresh spinach
1/2 cup fresh mushrooms
1 tablespoon stevia, raw honey or agave nectar
1 tablespoon apple cider vinegar

1 teaspoon baking soda
1 teaspoon baking powder
1 teaspoon ground white pepper (or black pepper)
1/2 teaspoon ground nutmeg
1/2 teaspoon dried basil

Directions

Preheat oven to 350 degrees F. Line muffin pan with paper liners or lightly coat with coconut oil. Heat medium pan over medium-high heat. Slice mushrooms and add to hot pan. Sauté about 3 minutes, then add spinach. Sauté until water evaporates, mushrooms are cooked through and spinach is wilted. Set aside. Beat eggs, sweetener and vinegar in medium mixing bowl with hand mixer or whisk until thick and frothy. Add sautéed veggies, almond flour, baking soda and powder and spices and mix until combined. Use ice cream scoop or tablespoon to pour batter into prepared muffin pan. Bake 15 - 20 minutes, until edges are golden brown and tops are firm. Remove muffins from oven and let cool about 5 minutes. Serve warm. Or allow to cool complete and serve temperature.

Serves: 12	Prep Time: 10 mins.	Cook Time: 15 mins.	
Calories: 30	Protein: 1.8g	Carbs: 2.1g	Fat: 1.7g

182. Cocoa Spice Pinwheel Cookies

Ingredients

2 cups almond flour
2 tablespoon stevia, raw honey or agave nectar
1 egg
1 teaspoon vanilla
1/2 teaspoon baking powder
1/4 teaspoon sea salt

Filling

2 tablespoons cocoa powder
2 tablespoons stevia, raw honey or agave nectar
2 teaspoons ground cinnamon
1 teaspoon ground black pepper
1/2 teaspoon vanilla

Directions

Preheat oven to 300 degrees F. Line sheet pan with parchment or baking mat. Prepare 2 additional sheets of parchment. Add flour, egg, sweetener, vanilla, baking powder and salt to medium bowl. Blend with wooden spoon, then knead with hand to form thick dough. Divide dough in half. Place half of dough in small mixing bowl. Add all Filling ingredients to bowl and mix until well combined. Roll out each half of dough separately on parchment sheets. Roll into equal rectangles. Place Filling rectangle on top of plain dough. Use parchment to help roll dough tightly along long edge into log. Use sharp knife to cut log into 1/4 round slices. Place cookies on prepared sheet pan and bake about 10 minutes, until edges are golden brown.
Switch off the oven and set to cool for 5 minutes. Serve warm. Or let cool completely and serve room temperature.

Serves: 12	Prep Time: 10 mins.	Cook Time: 10 mins.	
Calories: 38	Protein: 1g	Carbs: 7g	Fat: 1g

183. Rosemary Basil Scones

Ingredients

2 cups almond flour
1/3 cup arrowroot flour
1 egg
1/4 cup organic coconut oil
1/2 lemon
2 tablespoons stevia, orange juice, raw honey or agave nectar

2 teaspoons baking powder
2 sprigs fresh rosemary
5 - 6 large basil leaves (or 1 1/2 teaspoons dried basil)
1/2 teaspoon vanilla
1/2 teaspoon sea salt
1/4 cup hazelnuts (optional)

Directions

Preheat oven to 350 degrees F. Line sheet pan with parchment or coat with coconut oil. Whisk together flours, baking powder, salt and vanilla in large mixing bowl. Zest 1/2 lemon into small mixing bowl. Finely chop rosemary and chiffon fresh basil. Add herbs to bowl with egg and sweetener. Beat with hand mixer or whisk while slowly pouring in coconut oil. Add egg mixture to flour blend and mix until well combined. Chop and fold in hazelnuts (optional). Form dough into ball and place on sheet pan. Flatten to 1/2-inch-thick circle with hands. Cut into eight wedges with pizza cutter or sharp knife. Arrange at least 1 inch apart on sheet pan and bake for 20 - 25 minutes, or until edges are golden brown. Remove and let cool. Serve room temperature.

Serves: 8	Prep Time: 10 mins.	Cook Time: 25 mins.
Calories: 126	Protein: 1.9g	Carbs: 6.5g Fat: 10.8g

184. Apple Bread

Ingredients

2 cups coconut flour
1 cup almond flour
2 tablespoons tapioca flour (or arrowroot powder)
2 eggs
1 tart apple
1 sweet apple
1/2 cup unsweetened applesauce
1/4 cup coconut oil

1/4 cup stevia, raw honey or agave nectar
1 tablespoon baking soda
1 tablespoon apple cider vinegar
1 teaspoon ground cinnamon
1 teaspoon ground ginger
1 teaspoon sea salt
1/2 teaspoon white pepper

Directions

Preheat oven to 375 degrees F. Line 2 muffin pans with paper liners or coat with coconut oil. Peel, core and grate or dice apples, and place in small bowl. Pour vinegar and spices over apples. Toss to coat. In medium bowl, whisk eggs with hand mixer or whisk until light and thickened, about 2 minutes. Add applesauce, sweetener and coconut oil. Blend until combined. Mix in apples. Sift flours, baking soda and salt into apple mixture and mix until combined. Use ice cream scoop or tablespoon to scoop equal portions of batter into muffin pans until 2/3 - 3/4 full. Place in oven and bake for 15 - 20 minutes, or until golden brown and firm but springy to the touch. Switch the oven off and allow to cool for 5 minutes. Serve warm.

Serves: 24	Prep Time: 10 mins.	Cook Time: 20 mins.
Calories: 59	Protein: 1g	Carbs: 7.3g Fat: 3.2g

185. Pumpkin Coconut Bread

Ingredients

1 3/4 cups coconut flour
2 eggs
1/4 cup coconut oil
1/2 cup coconut milk
1/2 unsweetened applesauce
1/4 cup stevia, raw honey or agave nectar
15 oz (1 can) pumpkin puree

2 teaspoons baking soda
1 tablespoon ground cinnamon
1 teaspoon ground nutmeg
1 teaspoon sea salt
1/2 cup flaked coconut
1/4 cup pumpkin seeds
Water

Directions

Preheat oven to 350 degrees F. Coat square baking pan with coconut oil. Process eggs, coconut oil, coconut milk, applesauce and sweetener in food processor or blender until thick and lightened. Pour into medium mixing bowl. Mix in pumpkin puree and spices. Mix in flour, baking soda, flaked coconut and pumpkin seeds. Stir until combined. Pour batter into oiled baking pan. Bake 20 - 25 minutes, or until firm but springy in center. Serve warm or room temperature.

Serves: 12	Prep Time: 5 mins.	Cook Time: 25 mins.	
Calories: 272	Protein: 9.5g	Carbs: 28.2g	Fat: 14.7g

186. Fruit Parfait

Ingredients

¼ cup of chopped pineapple
½ kiwi chopped
1 banana sliced
½ cup of non-fat yogurt

2 tablespoons of high fiber cereal
2 tablespoons of coconut shredded sprinkle top with cinnamon

Directions

Mix all the fruit in a bowl together then put yogurt in another bowl put fruit mixture on top of yogurt, shredded coconut and cereal and top with some cinnamon.

Serves: 4	Prep Time: 10 mins.	Cook Time: 0 mins.	
Calories: 68	Protein: 3.1g	Carbs: 10.4g	Fat: 1.7g

187. Banana Chocolate Swirl Bread

Ingredients

1 tsp of vanilla extract
½ cup of buttermilk
½ teaspoon of salt
½ teaspoon of baking powder
¾ cup of whole wheat flour
2 large eggs

¼ cup of olive oil
2/ 3 cup of sugar substitute – coconut palm sugar
2 ripe bananas
2 ounces of bittersweet chocolate chopped
¾ cup of all-purpose flour

Directions

Preheat oven to 350 lightly dust 9 x 5 inch metal loaf pan with non-stick cooking spray then cover with flour shake off the excess. Put chocolate in bowl and place in the microwave at high for 30 seconds. Combine sugar substitute and bananas mash in bowl. Combine eggs and oil then combine your salt, baking powder and flours. Stir in buttermilk and vanilla. Stir 1 cup of batter into chocolate. Fill pan with half banana batter and half chocolate batter. Then repeat layering. Swirl with knife to mix them a little together to give you the swirl effect. Bake for about 45 minutes or until golden brown on top then allow to cool on wire rack.

Serves: 12	Prep Time: 10 mins.	Cook Time: 45 mins.	
Calories: 143	Protein: 2.7g	Carbs: 20.7g	Fat: 5.7g

188. Carrot Cup Cakes

Ingredients

¾ cup of whole wheat pastry flour
½ cup of all-purpose flour
¼ cup of fine salt
½ tsp of ground cinnamon pinch of nutmeg
½ cup of sugar substitute that can be used for baking and another
½ cup for frosting

¼ cup of olive oil
2 large eggs
1 ½ cups of finely shredded carrots
½ cup of natural applesauce
½ tsp of vanilla extract
½ cup of chopped

Directions

Preheat oven to 350-line 12 standard muffin cups with paper cupcake liners. Mix sugar substitute, eggs, oil. Add carrots, applesauce, and vanilla. Add dry ingredients mixing until combined stir in chopped walnuts put a few aside to put on top of cupcakes. Divide batter into muffin cups then bake for about 20 minutes transfer to wire rack. Beat together cream, zest, sugar substitute for frosting. Then frost cooled cupcakes adding the remaining walnuts on top of the cupcakes.

Serves: 12	Prep Time: 15 mins.	Cook Time: 20 mins.	
Calories: 236	Protein: 4g	Carbs: 10g	Fat: 16.7g

189. Pumpkin Parfait

Ingredients

1 cup pumpkin puree
1 package of instant sugar-free vanilla pudding
1 tsp of pumpkin spice

1 cup of evaporated milk
1 cup skim milk

Directions

Mix all ingredients in a bowl and blend well then put into parfait glasses and chill until set.

Serves: 1   **Prep Time: 10 mins.**   **Cook Time: 0 mins.**
Calories: 82   **Protein: 4.2g**   **Carbs: 5.2g**   **Fat: 5.5g**

190. Chocolate Pudding with Chia Seeds

Ingredients

2 cups unsweetened almond milk
1/2 cup chia seeds
1/4 cup natural creamy almond butter,

1/4 cup unsweetened cocoa powder
4 large dates, pitted and finely chopped
1 teaspoon pure vanilla extract

Directions

Place all ingredients into a bowl until thoroughly combined. Move bowl to refrigerator and chill pudding for 3 – 4 hours or overnight. Transfer pudding to blender or food processor and process until creamy. If pudding is too thick, thin it with a little more almond milk.

Serves: 4   **Prep Time: 10 mins.**   **Cook Time: 0 mins.**
Calories: 343   **Protein: 13g**   **Carbs: 29.3g**   **Fat: 22.1g**

191. Sautéed Apples

Ingredients

2 teaspoons butter, melted
1 granny smith apple, peeled, cored, and sliced

1/4 teaspoon cinnamon
1/4 teaspoon mace or nutmeg
pinch sea salt

Directions

Set a skillet on medium heat with your butter. Set your apple slices in your skillet evenly. Sprinkle with the salt, cinnamon and mace. Stir gently so that the apples are coated. Sauté for approximately 10 minutes, stirring occasionally, or until the apples have slightly softened. Serve warm. Try it with a splash of coconut milk and some extra cinnamon, if desired.

Serves: 1   **Prep Time: 10 mins.**   **Cook Time: 10 mins.**
Calories: 169   **Protein: 0.9g**   **Carbs: 23.5g**   **Fat: 8.2g**

192. Sweet Banana Shortbreads

Ingredients

1 cup coconut flour
2 overripe bananas
2 cage-free eggs
Honey, 1/4 cup, raw
coconut oil, 1/4 cup

1 tsp. baking powder
1/2 tsp. ground cinnamon
1/2 tsp. vanilla
1/2 tsp. of Celtic sea salt

Directions

Preheat oven to 350 degrees F. Line sheet pan with baking mat or lightly coat with coconut oil.
Add eggs to food processor or high-speed blender and process until light and fluffy, about 2 minutes. Peel and add bananas, sweetener, oil or butter, cinnamon and vanilla. Process until well combined. Add almond flour, baking powder and salt. Process until dough comes together. Roll dough into 12 balls and place on prepared sheet pan. Press to flatten. Set to bake for about 15 minutes, your edges should be golden. Switch off the oven and set to cool at least 5 minutes. Serve warm. Or transfer to wire rack to cool completely and serve room temperature.

Serves: 12	**Prep Time: 10 mins.**	**Cook Time: 30 mins.**
Calories: 104	**Protein: 1.9g**	**Carbs: 11.3g** **Fat: 6.3g**

193. Asian Orange Muffins

Ingredients

1 1/2 cups almond flour
2 eggs
1 1/2 cups grated carrot
1 tablespoon orange zest
coconut oil, 1/4 cup
Applesauce, 1/4 cup, unsweetened
orange juice, 1/2 cup

1 tablespoon grated fresh ginger
1 tablespoon ground ginger
1 tsp. vanilla
1 tsp. baking soda
1 tsp. baking powder
1/2 tsp. sea salt

Directions

Preheat oven to 350 degrees F. Line muffin pan with paper liners or coconut oil. Peel ginger. Grate ginger and carrots. In medium bowl beat eggs with hand mixer or whisk until light and a bit frothy. Add oil, applesauce, orange juice and zest. Beat well. Fold in carrots and ginger. Sift and stir in flour, baking soda and powder, spices and salt until combined. Use ice cream scoop or tablespoon to scoop batter into muffin tins, about 1/2 - 3/4 full. Bake 15 - 18 minutes, or until toothpick inserted into center comes out clean. Serve warm or room temperature.

Serves: 12	**Prep Time: 10 mins.**	**Cook Time: 15 mins.**
Calories: 78	**Protein: 1.8g**	**Carbs: 3.9g** **Fat: 6.3g**

194. Sage Sausage Buns

Ingredients

8 oz uncooked natural sage sausage

3/4 cup coconut flour

4 eggs

1/4 cup unsweetened applesauce

1/4 almond milk

1 teaspoon baking powder

2 tablespoons ground sage

1 tablespoon fresh basil

1 teaspoon ground white pepper (or black pepper)

1/2 teaspoon salt

Directions

Preheat oven to 350 degrees F. Coat muffin pan with coconut oil. Heat medium skillet over medium heat. Brown sausage in skillet for about 5 minutes, until half way cooked. Set aside and reserve leftover oil. While sausage browns, separate eggs. In large bowl, whisk egg whites to soft peaks with hand mixer or whisk. Add yolks, applesauce and almond milk. Mix until combined. Mince basil.

Sift flour, baking soda and salt into egg mixture. Add pepper, sage and basil. Stir to combine. Distribute par-cooked sausage evenly into each muffin pan cup. Use ice cream scoop or spoon to scoop batter on top of sausage. Fill each cup no more than 3/4 full. Baste with sausage dripping before placing in oven. Bake 15 - 20 minutes, or until tops are golden brown and firm to the touch. Turn out buns onto plate. Serve warm or room temperature.

Serves: 8	Prep Time: 10 mins.	Cook Time: 15 mins.	
Calories: 164	Protein: 7.8g	Carbs: 19.9g	Fat: 8.6g

195. Easy Biscuits

Ingredients

2 1/2 cups fine ground almond flour

2 eggs

1/4 cup coconut oil

1 teaspoon baking soda

1/2 teaspoon sea salt

1 tablespoon stevia, raw honey or agave nectar

Directions

Preheat oven to 350 degrees F. Line sheet pan with parchment paper. Combine salt, baking soda and almond flour in medium bowl. Separate egg whites into separate medium bowl, and yolk into small bowl. Beat egg whites to soft peaks with hand mixer or whisk. Mix yolks, oil and sweetener into whites. Mix wet ingredients into dry to form soft, solid dough. Roll dough into eight (8)1-inch thick round biscuits with hands. Place on parchment covered sheet pan and bake for 12 - 15 minutes, or until golden and firm on top. Serve warm.

Serves: 8	Prep Time: 5 mins.	Cook Time: 15 mins.	
Calories: 101	Protein: 2.3g	Carbs: 2.5g	Fat: 9.4g

196. Frontier Tortillas

Ingredients

2 tablespoons almond flour
1 1/2 tablespoons coconut flour
1/2 tablespoon flax meal (or ground chia seed)
2 eggs
1/4 cup water

2 tablespoons coconut oil
1/4 teaspoon baking powder
Extra water
Coconut oil (for cooking)

Directions

Lightly coat a skillet with coconut oil and set on medium heat to get hot. Whisk together eggs, coconut oil and 1/4 cup water in medium bowl. In another bowl, combine baking powder, chia seed, flax, almond flour and coconut flour. Pour the mixture slowly into your wet ingredients while whisking. If batter appears too thick to spread fairly thin in pan, add water 1 tablespoon at a time. Do not exceed 4 tablespoons.

Add 1/2 of batter into your hot oiled pan. Start moving your pan in a circular motion to allow your batter to spread thinly. Allow to cook for 2 minutes, your tortilla should be slightly golden. Flip over your tortilla and allow the other side to also cook for about 2 minutes. Transfer tortilla onto a paper towel or parchment. Fill warm tortillas with your favorite fillings and enjoy!

Serves: 2   **Prep Time: 5 mins.**   **Cook Time: 10 mins.**
Calories: 278   **Protein: 10.1g**   **Carbs: 5.9g**   **Fat: 24.1g**

197. Sweet Cherry Fig Newtons

Ingredients

Cookie Dough

1 1/2 cups almond flour

1/4 cup dried pitted dates

1/4 cup date butter (or agave or honey)

1/4 cup coconut oil (or cacao or coconut butter, melted)

1 teaspoon vanilla

1/4 teaspoon Celtic sea salt

Cherry Fig Filling

1/2 cup dried black mission figs

1/4 cup pitted cherries (fresh or thawed)

1/4 teaspoon ground ginger

Directions

Preheat oven to 350 degrees F. Line sheet pan with parchment or baking mat. For Cookie Dough, Add dried dates, date butter, and oil or melted butter to food processor or high-speed blender. Process until coarsely ground, about 1 - 2 minutes. Sift almond flour and salt into medium mixing bowl. Add date mixture to flour mixture and mix to combine. Set aside. For Filling, remove stems from figs and add to clean food processor or high-speed blender with cherries and ginger. Process until smooth mixture forms, about 2 minutes. Set aside.

Divide dough in half. Roll first half of dough into long, thin rectangle about 1/4-inch-thick between 2 parchment sheets. Spread 1/2 of Cherry Fig Filling along one side of the dough, long-ways. Use parchment to fold dough in half along long edge so plain dough covers side with Cherry Fig Filling. Dough should resemble flattened log. Press edges of dough together for tight seal. Place on prepared sheet pan. Repeat with remaining Cookie Dough and Cherry Fig Filling. Set to bake for about 15 minutes, your edges should be golden brown. Switch the oven off and allow to cool for 5 minutes. Then slice logs into 2-inch cookies. Serve immediately.

Serves: 12   Prep Time: 10 mins.   Cook Time: 15 mins.

Calories: 102   Protein: 0.5g   Carbs: 7.7g   Fat: 8.1g

198. Walnut Raisin Cookies

Ingredients

1 1/4 cups almond flour
1 cage-free egg
1/4 cup coconut oil (or cacao or coconut butter)
1/4 cup raw honey (or agave or date butter)
1/4 cup cashew butter

1/2 cup walnuts
1/4 cup raisins
1 teaspoon baking powder
1 teaspoon vanilla
1/4 teaspoon Celtic sea salt

Directions

Preheat oven to 350 degrees F. Line sheet pan with parchment or baking mat. Sift flour, baking powder and salt into medium mixing bowl. Beat with whisk or hand mixer to lighten. Add egg, oil or butter, sweetener, cashew butter, vanilla and salt. Mix well to form dough. Chop walnuts and add to bowl with raisins. Mix to combine. Shape dough into 12 balls and place onto prepared baking sheet. Flatten slightly with hand or spatula. Place in oven and bake 10 - 15 minutes, until golden brown along edges. Remove from oven and let cool 5 minutes. Serve warm. Or transfer to wire rack to cool completely and serve room temperature.

Serves: 12   **Prep Time: 10 mins.**   **Cook Time: 15 mins.**
Calories: 129   **Protein: 1.3g**   **Carbs: 6.5g**   **Fat: 11.4g**

199. Rainbow Trifle with Whipped Cream

Ingredients

1 cup RED fruit, sliced (sliced strawberries, raspberries, watermelon)
1 cup ORANGE fruit (nectarines, cantaloupe)
1 cup YELLOW fruit (pineapple, mango)
1 cup GREEN fruit (kiwi, green grapes, honeydew)
1 cup BLUE fruit (blueberries)

1 cup PURPLE fruit (purple grapes, blackberries)
1 can full-fat coconut milk, refrigerated
1 teaspoon ground ginger
1 teaspoon ground cinnamon
1 date, unsweetened

Directions

Take the coconut milk out of the refrigerator. Spoon the thick coconut "cream" out of the can into a blender jar. Add the banana, ginger, cinnamon, and date to the blender jar. Process until combined. In a large glass bowl, mix the fruits. Serve the fruits with the coconut-banana cream spooned on top.

Serves: 6-8   **Prep Time: 10 mins.**   **Cook Time: 0 mins.**
Calories: 132   **Protein: 1.2g**   **Carbs: 34g**   **Fat: 0.2g**

200. Butter Pecan Frozen Custard

Ingredients

13 oz (1 can) full-fat coconut milk
4 oz lite coconut milk (or water)
5 cage-free egg yolks
2 - 4 tablespoons ghee (or cacao or coconut butter)

1/4 cup raw honey (or agave, date butte or stevia)
1/2 cup chopped pecans
1 teaspoon vanilla

Directions

Freeze ice cream maker canister overnight to make sure it is cold enough. Heat medium pan over medium heat. Chop pecans and add to hot pan. Toasted until lightly golden and aromatic, about 5 minutes. Remove from pan and set aside. Add butter, coconut milk and water, if using, to hot pan. When mixture is warmed, but not hot, whisk in egg yolks, sweetener and vanilla. Continue whisking until thickened, about 5 minutes. Turn on ice cream maker first, then carefully pour in coconut milk mixture as ice cream maker paddle rotates. Freeze mixture about 5 minutes. Sprinkle toasted pecans into ice cream maker as mixture freezes and thickens. Freeze mixture another 10 - 15 minutes. Then transfer to serving dish. Serve immediately. Or store in air tight container in freezer.

Serves: 4   Prep Time: 15 mins.   Cook Time: 25 mins.
Calories: 169   Protein: 0.9g   Carbs: 23.5g   Fat: 8.2g

201. Cherry Nut Rugelach

Ingredients

Crust

2 cups almond flour

2 cage-free eggs

2 tablespoons coconut oil

2 tablespoons cacao butter, melted (or full-fat coconut milk)

2 tablespoons raw honey (or agave or date butter)

1 teaspoon baking powder

1/2 teaspoon baking soda

1/2 teaspoon vanilla

1/4 teaspoon ground cinnamon

1/4 teaspoon ground ginger

1/4 teaspoon Celtic sea salt

Filling

1/2 cup dried cherries

1/2 cup walnuts

1/2 cup raw honey (or agave or date butter)

2 tablespoons ghee, melted (or cacao or coconut butter, melted)

1/2 teaspoon cinnamon

1/2 teaspoon ginger

Pinch Celtic sea salt

Splash of Brandy (optional)

Directions

For Crust, sift almond flour into medium mixing bowl. Add baking soda and powder, vanilla, cinnamon, ginger and salt. Whisk eggs and sweetener in small mixing bowl, then add to flour mixture and combine. Slowly add coconut oil and cacao butter or coconut milk until malleable dough comes together. Roll in plastic wrap or wrap tightly in parchment and refrigerate for 15 minutes.

Preheat oven to 325 degrees F. Line sheet pan with parchment or baking mat. Cover cutting board with parchment. Heat medium pan over medium heat. For Filling, add walnuts to dry hot pan and toast about 2 minutes, stirring frequently. Add ghee, sweetener, cherries, salt, spices and splash of Brandy (optional) to walnuts. Stir while cooking until heated through. Remove from heat and set aside to cool. Remove dough from refrigerator.

Roll dough out on parchment covered cutting board to about 1/4-inch-thick rectangle with rolling pin. Spread Filling over dough. Use sharp knife or pizza cutter to cut dough into about 12 rectangles. Roll up dough pieces and arrange on prepared sheet pan. Bake 20 - 25 minutes, until dough is golden brown and cooked through. Switch off the oven and allow to cool for 5 minutes. Serve warm.

Serves: 12   **Prep Time: 25 mins.**   **Cook Time: 25 mins.**

Calories: 158   **Protein: 2.2g**   **Carbs: 16.3g**   **Fat: 10.2g**

202. Healthy Pineapple Coconut Cake

Ingredients

6 cage-free eggs
3/4 cup coconut flour
1 cup flaked coconut
1 1/2 cups pineapple (diced)
1/2 cup raw honey (or agave or date butter)

1/2 cup coconut oil (or cacao or coconut butter, melted)
1 teaspoon baking soda
1 teaspoon baking powder
1 teaspoon vanilla
1/2 teaspoon Celtic sea salt

Directions

Preheat oven to 350 degrees F. Lightly coat square or rectangular baking dish with coconut oil. Add eggs to food processor or high-speed blender. Process until pale and lightened, about 2 minutes. Add flour, coconut, pineapple, sweetener, oil or butter, baking soda, baking powder, vanilla and salt. Blend to get it combined well, about 1 - 2 minutes. Pour batter into prepared baking dish and bake about 45 minutes, until golden brown and firm in the center. Switch off the oven and set to cool about 10 minutes. Slice and serve warm. Or let cool completely and serve room temperature.

Serves: 12   Prep Time: 10 mins.   Cook Time: 45 mins.
Calories: 202   Protein: 5g   Carbs: 18.4g   Fat: 13g

203. Lemon Bundt Cake

Ingredients

6 cage-free eggs
1 cup almond flour
3 large lemons
1/2 cup raw honey (or agave or date butter)

1/4 cup coconut oil (cacao or coconut butter, melted)
2 teaspoons baking soda
1 teaspoon vanilla
1/2 teaspoon Celtic sea salt

Directions

Preheat oven to 350 degrees F. Coat Bundt pan with coconut oil. Add eggs to food processor or high-speed blender. Process until pale and lightened, about 2 minutes. Zest 1 lemon, then juice all lemons into processor. Add flour, sweetener, oil or butter, baking soda, vanilla and salt. Blend until combined. Pour batter into prepared Bundt pan and bake about 45 minutes, until golden brown and toothpick inserted halfway between center and edge of pan comes out clean. Remove oven and let cool 15 minutes. Turn cake out onto serving dish. Slice and serve warm.

Serves: 12   Prep Time: 15 mins.   Cook Time: 45 mins.
Calories: 146   Protein: 4.3g   Carbs: 13g   Fat: 8.7g

204. Indian Almond Balls

Ingredients

1 1/2 cup almond flour
1/2 cup almond butter
1/4 cup dried pitted dates
2 tablespoons raw honey (or agave or stevia)
1 tablespoon lemon juice
1 teaspoon lemon zest

1/2 teaspoon ground cardamom (optional)
1/4 teaspoon Celtic sea salt

Topping

1/2 cup pistachios
1/4 -1/3 cup shredded or flaked coconut

Directions

For Topping, add pistachios to food processor or high-speed blender. Process until finely ground, about 1 minute. Add to shallow dish with coconut and mix to combine. Set aside. Add almond flour, almond butter, dates, sweetener, salt and cardamom (optional) to clean food processor or high-speed blender. Zest then juice lemon into processor. Blend to ground and form a tacky dough, about 3 minutes. Shape dough into golf ball sized rounds. Place in Topping and roll to coat. Gently press with palms to secure pistachio flour and coconut on dough. Transfer to serving dish and serve room temperature.

Serves: 12	Prep Time: 10 mins.	Cook Time: 10 mins.
Calories: 119	Protein: 1.3g	Carbs: 7g Fat: 10.1g

205. Simple Chinese Moon Cakes

Ingredients

2/3 cup coconut flour
2 cage-free egg yolks
1/2 cup ghee (or cacao or coconut butter)
1/4 cup date butter (or agave or raw honey)

Filling

1 cup dried fruit (apricots, strawberries, blueberries, etc.)
Water

Directions

Preheat oven to 375 degrees F. Cover sheet pan with parchment or baking mat. In medium mixing bowl, cream ghee, sweetener and 1 egg yolk with hand mixer or wooden spoon. Add flour and mix until dough comes together. Wrap dough in plastic wrap or parchment and refrigerate 30 minutes. For Filling, add dried apricots to clean food processor or high-speed blender. Process until thick jam forms, about 1 - 2 minutes. Add enough water to reach desired consistency.

Remove dough from refrigerator. Form 24 balls from dough and place on prepared sheet pan. Press thumb into each ball to create indent. Fill each indent with Filling. Add remaining egg yolk and 1 teaspoon water to small mixing bowl and brush each Moon Cake with egg wash. Set to bake for about 20 minutes, your edges should be slightly browned. Switch the oven off and allow to cool for 5 minutes. Serve warm.

Serves: 12	Prep Time: 10 mins.	Cook Time: 10 mins.
Calories: 147	Protein: 1g	Carbs: 7.4g Fat: 13.2g

Interested in becoming a master chef? ;)

If you liked the recipes in this book, then you might be interested in the following books.

Dash Slow Cooker Cookbook
Link to Amazon:
https://amzn.to/2XK6XYW

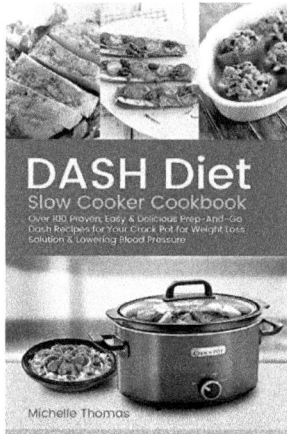

Anti-Inflammatory Diet Instant Pot
Cookbook Link to Amazon:
https://amzn.to/2TrBkoL

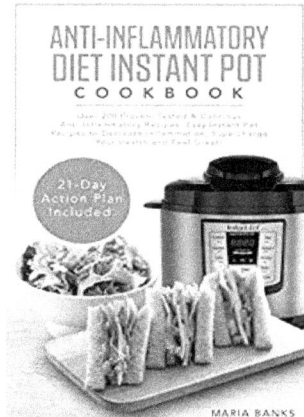

Prediabetes Cookbook
Link to Amazon:
https://amzn.to/2XMtC7i

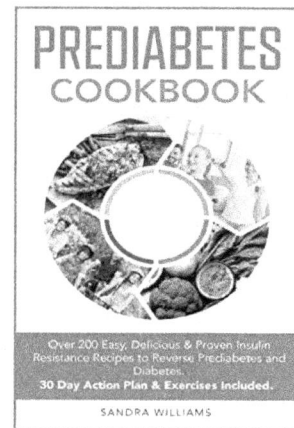

Mind Diet Cookbook
Link to Amazon:
https://amzn.to/2Ttctke

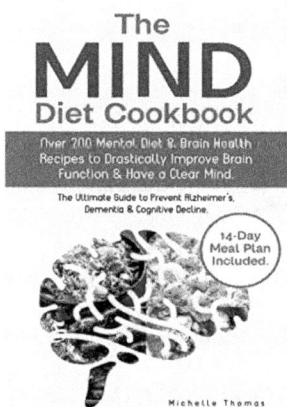

Dash Cookbook
Link to Amazon:
https://amzn.to/2HgXGly

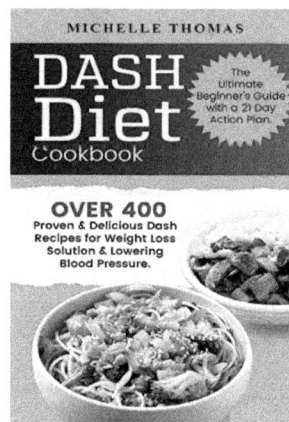

Keto Fat Bombs Cookbook
Link to Amazon:
https://amzn.to/2Cb7t9A

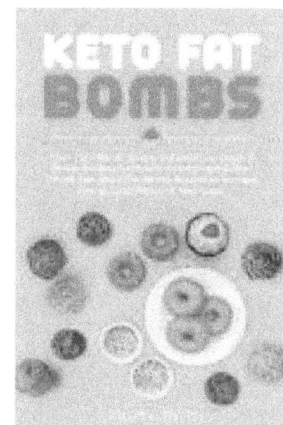

Type 2 Diabetes Cookbook
Link to Amazon:
https://amzn.to/2Uqzzo8

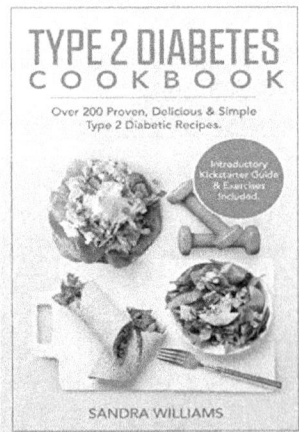

PCOS Cookbook
Link to Amazon:
https://amzn.to/2tYbOsc

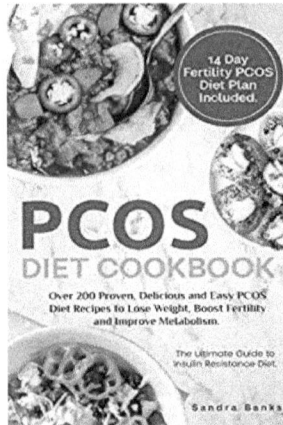

Lectin Free Diet Cookbook
Link to Amazon:
https://amzn.to/2XMqxUI

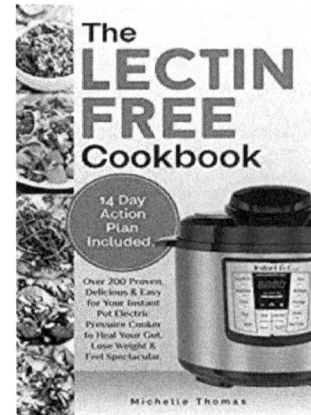

Dukan Diet Cookbook
Link to Amazon:
https://amzn.to/2EPmXjO

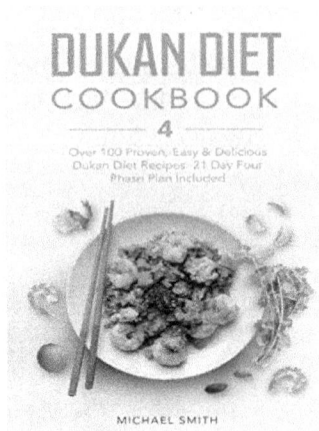

Mini Instant Pot Cookbook
Link to Amazon:
https://amzn.to/2NQXo68

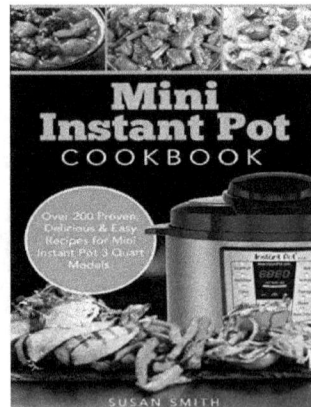

We sincerely hope you enjoyed the recipes.

If you feel like we could improve the cookbook please email us at info@limitlessrecipes.com and we'll make sure to get back to you.

We have a big passion for cooking and we love writing cookbooks but quite often it's pretty hard to compete with all the big publishing companies out there. Reviews really help us and we would appreciate it if you could take a minute and leave a review of the book.

If you could take one minute to leave a review, we would really appreciate that.

You can also leave a review by following these 3 steps:
1. Go to the product page
2. Scroll down and on the left side click 'Write customer review'
3. Write a review and click 'Submit'

Thank you, it really means a lot. Who's amazing? You are!

Conclusion

Thank you for sticking with us all the way to the end! We hope we were able to set you on the right path to selecting and preparing a delicious meal with to help with your weight loss battle using these Pre-Diabetes recipes whether it be for you, a relative or a close friend.

So, what happens next?

Keep practicing and explore new and exciting meals from the Pre-Diabetes diet. Mix and match the delicious recipes presented in this book to come up with your favorite Pre-Diabetes diet meals then share them with your friends, and family!

Once again, thank you for allowing us to help you on this Pre - Diabetes diet journey, and feel free to leave us a positive review if you like what you read through.

Until next time … best of luck!

CPSIA information can be obtained
at www.ICGtesting.com
Printed in the USA
LVHW060731270720
661604LV00016B/897

9 781729 657614